The
Science
of
Sex

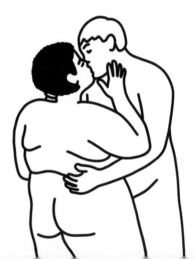

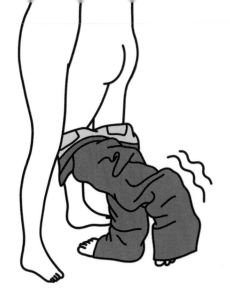

The Science of Sex

KATE MOYLE

ILLUSTRATED BY JOCELYN COVARRUBIAS

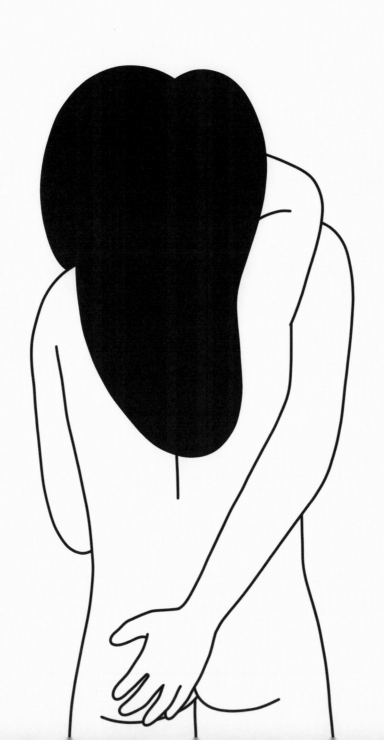

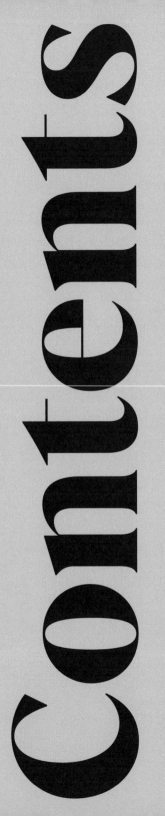

Contents

Talking
about sex

I've never met a person who didn't have a question about sex. One of the main parts of my job as a psychosexual therapist is to help people find the answers that are right for them.

I've always been fascinated as to why the word "sex" evokes a certain reaction from people – a shift in body language, a change in the tone of voice – conversations feel like they've turned a corner once the topic is brought up. Even in 2023, saying you're a psychosexual therapist raises eyebrows. Equally, I've wondered why so much of the focus of sex education is about the doing, when sex can't be detached from our psychology and emotions – even when it's with someone we're not emotionally attached to.

Sex feels like an area where we're expected to be experts without the process of becoming one - questioning, learning, trial and error. Although a subjective experience, sex is also a skill to be learnt, but we don't have adequate teaching, leaving many worrying they're somehow failing at sex.

Having said all of this, we're in a time of huge change and development sexually. The sexual wellness industry is booming. New ventures are constantly launching – with a focus on inclusivity rather than just heteronormative sex – to help people improve their sexual education, pleasure, confidence, and wellbeing. Products such as lubricants and sex toys have migrated from dark corners onto high street shelves, normalizing sex alongside other areas of health and wellbeing. The funding and research being pumped into the industry are leading to developments that aim to improve sex for many.

Sex is both simple and a conundrum.

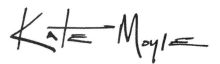

Sex is largely about our relationship with ourselves, much of which is rooted in our identity. Accordingly, this book uses inclusive terminology. Alongside the terms women and men, it refers to people with a vagina, vulva, or clitoris, people with a penis, and those assigned female/male at birth (AFAB/AMAB) – the language considered most inclusive at the time of writing. When quoting studies, we've adopted the language of the original research because many published studies don't specify further identifying information. This means it's not always clear exactly who is covered by a statistic, but we hope that the studies we've quoted still give an insight into a variety of experiences and opinions on sex.

No book could fit in every question or have every answer about sex, simply because human diversity means that one person could never talk about all there is to know. I see this subjectivity in my practice as each person I work with teaches me something new. Perhaps the most important thing to come out of reading this book will be to question yourself. What do you know about sex? Where did that come from? Does it enable you to fulfil your sexual potential, and if not, are you open to finding out how you can change your relationship with sex for the better? I hope this book sparks your curiosity.

Kate Moyle

Sex
education

Our sex education starts earlier than we think, and is in both the said and the unsaid. As well as the often inadequate sex education we receive at school, we absorb messages about sex from observing communication and touch in others; and from noticing the reaction of those around us, and our own sense of embarrassment, when presented with the subject unexpectedly. How we experience desire, our bodies' reactions, and the emotions we have around sex, all inform us, too. When sex education is good, messages around sex are positive; we embrace sexual diversity and sex becomes a normalized part of our health and wellbeing.

A brief history of sex

Sex is as old as time, but our approach to human sexuality has constantly evolved. Critical points throughout our sexual history have influenced the landscape of our sex lives today.

EVOLUTION OF SEX TOYS

The use of sex toys is documented over thousands of years, with reports of dildos used in Ancient Greece. In the early **1880s**, a Dr Granville patented the first vibrator.

THE USE OF CONDOMS

These are thought to date back thousands of years, with versions made from material such as animal bladders and skins, tortoiseshell, thin leather, and tied linen. A huge step forward came in the **1830s** with the invention by US chemist Charles Goodyear of vulcanized rubber condoms. By the 1920s, manufacturing advances saw the introduction of thinner, stronger latex condoms, whose use became widespread.

THE ADVENT OF MODERN SEX RESEARCH

In **1947**, Dr Alfred Kinsey, an American biologist and sexologist, founded the Institute For Sex Research. He went on to publish two widely acclaimed books, The Kinsey Reports *Sexual Behavior in the Human Male* (1948) and *Sexual Behavior in the Human Female* (1953), which challenged conventional beliefs about sexuality.

PORNOGRAPHY THROUGH TIME

Erotic depictions of desire and sex have been documented across different cultures throughout history – in cave wall carvings, art, drawings, writing, sculpture, and music. Today, pornography's most mainstream format is on film and camera, developing in line with fast-paced advances in technology and the internet.

THE *KAMA SUTRA*

This ancient illustrated Sanskrit book from India, dated **400BCE– 200CE**, is famous for detailing a variety of explorative and creative sex positions. It also examined desire, intimacy, sexuality, and love.

400BCE–200CE   1800   **1830**   1900   1947

A UK study found that between 2015 and 2019, 32% of couples met online.

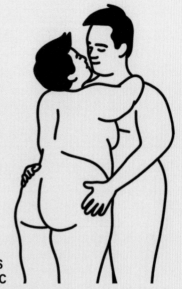

CONTINUED RESEARCH INTO SEXUALITY

In the late **1950s**, William Masters and Virginia Johnson pioneered research into human sexuality via the direct observation of human subjects. They measured anatomical and physiological sexual responses in laboratory settings. Their research played a huge part in our understanding of our sexual responses and started the conversation around our triggers for arousal and how sexual dysfunction or problems can occur.

INTRODUCTION OF THE PILL

In **1960**, the US Food and Drug Administration (FDA) approved the world's first commercially available birth control pill. In the UK, the pill was initially available for married women only, though it became available for all in 1967. The accessibility of the contraceptive pill led to the first sexual revolution, offering reproductive freedom and choice.

FIRST WOMEN'S SEX SHOP

In **1974**, Dell Williams opened the first women's sex shop – Eve's Garden in New York, USA.

HIV/AIDS EPIDEMIC

In **1981**, the US had the first official reporting of acquired immune deficiency syndrome (AIDS), caused by the human immunodeficiency virus (HIV) and, at least at first, massively impacting the gay male community. In 1999, the WHO announced it the fourth leading cause of death worldwide, and the number one cause of death in Africa.

VIAGRA APPROVED

In **1998**, the FDA approved the use of the drug Viagra to treat erectile dysfunction.

THE ADVENT OF ONLINE DATING

In **1995**, the first online dating site, Match.com, revolutionized how partners could meet. As smartphones became more commonly used, online dating became widely accessible. In **2009**, the gay and bisexual dating app Grindr was launched; in **2012**, Tinder introduced the concept of "swipe right" for matches. In **2018**, 93 out of 1,000 couples in *The Times'* wedding announcement column that year met online.

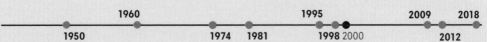

1950 · 1960 · 1974 · 1981 · 1995 · 1998 · 2000 · 2009 · 2012 · 2018

What is **sex?**

Often, sex is defined as an act that involves penetration. However, this view can be reductive, heteronormative, and focuses on one part of sex while ignoring much of what makes sex pleasurable.

Many of us accept the definition of sex that we're commonly taught – that it's something physical and biological with a reproductive focus based around intercourse, which is defined as putting a penis into a vagina (PIV). However, using the terms "sex" and "intercourse" interchangeably elevates intercourse to "real sex" and excludes other sexual practices we enjoy, or implies that somehow these are lesser.

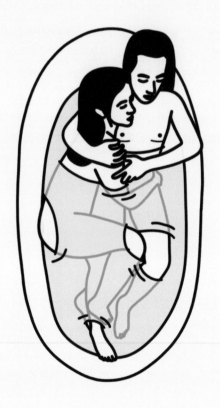

A problematic definition

When we focus on PIV sex, we fail to acknowledge relationships where there isn't both a penis and a vagina, and de-prioritize the sexual pleasure of those with a preference for other sexual expressions or who aren't physically able to have penetrative sex. This definition of sex also raises questions such as, "When you enjoy non-penetrative pleasure with your partner, doesn't that count as sex?"

Limiting the definition of sex to intercourse not only excludes certain groups and practices, it can also create pressure to adhere to a sexual model that might not work for us – in turn potentially capping our ability to experience sexual pleasure, connection, satisfaction, and fun. For example, when we feel that sex must include intercourse, this could mean we persevere with sex that isn't comfortable; or it might lead to problems such as performance anxiety and other sexual dysfunctions (see pp.118–123). The result is that we can end up having a sexual experience that feels negative, which in turn can affect our desire, relationships, intimacy, and level of self-acceptance. Ultimately, this can lead to feelings of shame around sex (see p.32).

Rewriting our sexual narrative

While intercourse plays a big role in many people's sex lives, it is in fact just one form of sexual expression. Thinking about the language we use around sex can help us start to re-examine our experiences. For example, the word "foreplay" suggests that this is something that happens first, before the main event, so sex becomes a linear, goal-oriented event. If, instead, we reframe this as "non-penetrative sex", we begin to understand that there are so many different ways we can enjoy sexual experiences. We

Being open to everything that sex can be helps us enjoy it to its fullest.

can embrace a more circular model of sex, where exploration is the focus and sex isn't goal-oriented (see p.130).

Sex involves our bodies, minds, and emotions, and the act of sex is co-created between those involved. When we think about the meaning and definition of sex as being based on what it gives us, rather than just its mechanics, our sexual world greatly expands. We can start to examine where our thoughts about what sex means originated, whether we see these thoughts as fixed or fluid, and how changing our definition of sex might change how we think, feel about, and have sex.

Is sex just
physical?

Approaching sex as a purely physical act is highly reductive and only goes so far in explaining what's going on when we have sex.

As well as being a physical experience, sex also involves us at a social and emotional level.

The full picture

Our sex lives involve us biologically, psychologically, and socially. Considering sex from just one of these perspectives doesn't give us a full understanding of our sexual experiences. In sexology – the scientific study of human sexuality – the biopsychosocial model is held as a gold standard for comprehending human sexuality. This sex positive approach deems a person's sexual expression as valid and meaningful, based on their individual context. It celebrates diversity and difference, rather than measuring individuals against a "norm", which can induce feelings of shame if we feel we aren't meeting an acceptable standard.

An interrelated response

Social and cultural messaging can affect us mentally and physically, as shown opposite. In the context of sex, an example is our response to stress. Stress is influenced by our social context, which can decide whether or not we focus on and respond to a stressor. If we do, the body's stress response is activated – blood pressure rises, the stress hormones adrenaline and cortisol are released, and heart rate and breathing quicken. This interruption to sexual arousal, which for many is stressful in itself, continues the relationship between stress and sex.

Sex is biological, psychological, and social. Understanding how these elements interconnect and influence each other is a key element of sexology.

Biology involves the brain and body. Neural activity triggers the release of neurochemicals that induce a physiological response; this in turn helps or hinders arousal.

Our sexual expression is individual, reflecting our physical, emotional, and social reality.

Social context, in terms of our society and culture, impacts how we respond psychologically to a stressor. Our context means we either maintain a physiological response, for example to stress, or complete the stress cycle, allowing arousal to continue.

Psychology involves our feelings as we assess the relevance of events. If a psychological stressor interferes with our ability to focus on sex, this can interrupt the physical arousal process.

Is sex good for our health?

Sex is much more than a simple act – it's intertwined with so many parts of our lives. Understanding its effects on body and mind helps us appreciate its benefits for our health and wellbeing.

A physical boost

Sexual activity is a physical exertion that acts as a form of aerobic exercise. During sex, our heart rate, breathing, and blood flow increase and we burn calories. The act of sex also makes us feel tired, promoting restful sleep that allows the body to recuperate.

An antidote to stress

Chronic stress can have a negative impact on our sex lives. For some people, sex itself can be a stressor, evidencing the bidirectional relationship between sex and our psychological and emotional wellbeing. However, for others, sex acts as a form of stress relief as they enjoy the mood-boosting effects of the neurochemicals oxytocin, dopamine, and endorphins, released during sex. Endorphins also act as a natural form of pain relief, easing the mental and physical impacts of stress. The beneficial effects of these neurochemicals can create a positive loop, boosting our desire and overall motivation for sex.

Research also reveals that intimacy offers a form of stress relief, buffering psycho-biological stress – which affects mind and body – and lowering levels of the stress hormone cortisol. Sex can also communicate the emotional support of a partner, which in turn helps us to manage our own emotional response to stress.

During orgasm, the additional surge of oxytocin we receive, as well as the release of prolactin, promote restful sleep. This also helps to counter the disturbed sleep associated with stress and in turn increase our resilience to stress.

A means of self-care

The surge of dopamine in our brain's reward pathways (see p.56) that we experience during sex is a key source of pleasure, which in itself is a form of self-care.

The feelings we enjoy during sex also help us build a positive narrative around our bodies and the pleasure they can offer, which in turn supports our sexual wellbeing. Pleasure also provides a mental release, allowing us to escape everyday concerns and focus completely on ourselves.

Closer connections

Part of the reason why sex can improve our wellbeing can be attributed to the ability of touch and physical intimacy between partners to create a deeper sense of connection. Physiologically, touch triggers the release of the bonding hormone, oxytocin, so when we explore each other's bodies, the release of this chemical helps us feel closer to our partners. We may also experience vulnerability, which can enhance connections further (see p.143).

Sex is a uniquely shared experience and is never the same with different partners. While some, such as asexual people (see p.36), feel they don't need sex to enjoy closeness, for others, sex offers an intimate way of getting to know another person in a different way to non-sexual relationships.

Increased self-confidence

Psychologically, positive sexual experiences and feeling desired by a partner can boost our sexual self-esteem and self-confidence. For many, the feeling of being wanted is extremely erotic and sexually motivating.

Self-exploration and pleasure also play a key role in learning about yourself and your preferences, providing a form of self-sex education. When we get to know our own bodies and enjoy the stand-alone benefits of sensual and sexual pleasure, we can also feel more confident introducing a partner to what we enjoy.

One study showed that 95% of men in heterosexual relationships said that feeling desired was important to their sexual experience.

Are **labels** for sexuality and gender helpful?

The labels we give ourselves, or that others give us, can hold meaning and power in our lives. Importantly, a label isn't the whole picture.

We use labels to describe a diverse range of sexual orientations and gender identities. How much or how little we identify with one or more labels is about our own identity, and whether we feel a sense of ownership and alignment with a label.

How labels can make us feel

Some find a label provides a place of safety and belonging. They may feel it gives them a feeling of being part of a community where they can express themselves. For others, a label can feel constraining, or not the right fit; they may find it creates a sense of separation and that assumptions may be made about them.

In terms of sexuality, or sexual orientation (see opposite), many are happy with a single label, while for others, sexuality is nuanced. In 1948, sexologist Dr Alfred Kinsey published *Sexual Behaviour In The Human Male*, which challenged the idea that sexuality was binary and people were, in the words of his research, strictly homosexual, bisexual, or heterosexual (see p.186). His research found that while some identified with binary labels – for example,

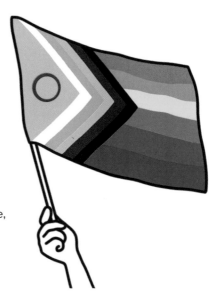

We rarely use one identifying label as humans are so multidimensional.

heterosexual or gay – for many, labels were limiting, as sexual behaviours, thoughts, and feelings were fluid over time.

Gender labels can also feel limiting, or not right, for some people. For example, transgender people feel that the gender label they grew up with doesn't align with who they know themselves to be. Acceptance for them may involve embracing a new label. For those who experience gender dysphoria, feeling a mismatch between their sex assigned at birth and their gender identity can create unease with labels.

A question of context

As well as being used to celebrate, labels can be used to attack; and social and legal contexts can influence how some express themselves. For example, discrimination – and sometimes threats – towards certain groups can mean some feel it's unsafe to express who they are publicly.

HOW LABELS HAVE EVOLVED

The terms we use to express gender (our socially constructed identities) and sexual orientation (how we experience sexual attraction) have broadened. Today we recognize a far wider expression of identities that moves away from binary descriptions.

- A transgender person is someone whose gender identity doesn't align with the sex they were assigned at birth.
- Non-binary people may describe themselves as agender (no gender), bigender (two genders), genderfluid (non-static gender), or other terms.
- The term pansexuality describes someone who feels attraction without noticing gender.
- Being asexual and/or aromantic, describes not feeling a sexual attraction to, or romantic interest in, others (see p.36).
- Demisexuals feel attraction only where there's an emotional connection.
- An emerging sexual orientation is digisexuality, which has developed alongside our increasing reliance on technology as part of our lives. This describes those who are sexually and/or romantically attracted to others through technology and devices, as well as people who enjoy sex with devices without another human interacting, for example, via virtual reality.
- The term queer can mean different things to different people. It can describe not identifying with heterosexual or cisgender norms, reflecting sexuality and gender as being on a spectrum. Many have reclaimed it after a history of use as a derogatory term.

How do I set sexual boundaries?

Our personal boundaries indicate how we want to be treated. They can be sexual, emotional, or physical, and we establish them to respect our own and others' values, limits, needs, and wants.

How we manage boundaries should be based on a model of respect for our differences.

The three "C"s

Setting out boundaries is critical when it comes to sex and intimacy and requires clear dialogue between ourselves and our partners. The three "C"s – **consent, communication, and curiosity** – are our cornerstones when establishing what we want and don't want.

Consent is something we practise constantly in our daily lives, and when it comes to sex it's critical and non-negotiable. The legal age of consent – when someone can legally agree to taking part in a sexual act – varies in different territories. Beyond this, personal consent is about freedom and choice – what we're happy to do when we agree to a sexual experience with a partner. Crucially, consent can be withdrawn or modified at any point.

Communication is how we exchange information on boundaries and can be both verbal and non-verbal, for example, by guiding your partner's hand to a part of your body. Communication is the way we understand each other so its success is key. Without it, we base our understanding of others on assumptions and our own perspective.

Curiosity is the desire to learn. It helps us to understand others and encourages us to be open-minded to another's needs and explore why certain boundaries are important to them. It also helps us to explore and understand our own wants and needs.

Working it out

Establishing boundaries starts with recognizing what's important to you, and appreciating that a partner, or partners, will have their own boundaries. Consider the following:

- **To explore sex safely** with a partner, you don't have to be perfectly sexually aligned. It's not unusual for partners to have differing sexual preferences and desires.
- **Think about big concepts**, such as respect and mutual feelings – not just the specifics of sex, which can be easier to hone in on.
- **Talk about what you're comfortable** doing, and what you might be comfortable trying, if and when you feel like it.

- **Exploring your own body** in your own time can help you identify what you like and don't like on your own terms. This in turn can help you clarify what you like without pressure or expectation from a partner.
- **Miscommunication** and misunderstanding can happen. It's helpful to work out how to manage these confidently when they occur.
- **Preferences can shift**, for example, as you get to know a partner. Regularly checking in with each other will help ensure you're both aware if something has changed.
- **If you notice your boundaries** are being pushed, say so. Consent and communication aren't about coercion. Examples of coercion include someone asking you to do something repeatedly until you say "yes"; and being given drugs and alcohol that impair communication. Phrases such as, "If you loved me you'd have sex"; "Everyone else is having sex"; "If we don't have sex, I'll tell others we did anyway"; and "If you don't do x, I'll do y" are also forms of coercion. Removing a condom during sex when consent was given on the basis of wearing one, known as "stealthing", is illegal in some countries, including the UK, and is seen as an abuse of consent.

- **Giving and receiving consent** can be expressed in a variety of ways:

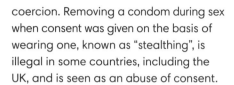

That feels really good – can we just take it slowly.

How do you like to be touched?

Do you want to carry on?

Would you like it if I did that?

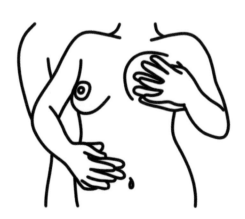

Do our **thoughts** affect sex?

Our self-reflective human nature means we constantly question ourselves. Working out how to navigate our thoughts about sex can help us address issues.

How we think about sex matters, as our thoughts translate our experiences and make sense of them. The brain's frontal lobe is the area that governs our thought processes. As our emotional and personality control centre, it plays a critical role in social interactions, as well as in our communicating, cognitive skills, emotional expression, and judgment. As with all our thought processes, how we think about sex is therefore multidimensional.

Reflective thinking

Our complex thought processes mean that we think about and reflect on our own thinking and learning – a concept known as metacognition. So when we have a sexual thought, fantasy, or a physical arousal response, these can trigger self-reflective thoughts. We may question, for example, why something is arousing us; or whether it's normal to have a certain thought and if other people have similar ones. This process can become problematic if we feel that the answers reflect negatively on us and that somehow we aren't fitting into a perceived sexual "norm". This can create stress, anxiety, and feelings of shame. As a result, we may try to shape our sex lives to fit in with what we think is acceptable, rather than follow our genuine wants and desires.

Positive thinking

When we accept self-questioning thoughts with less self-criticism, we can build awareness of the underlying factors that may have led to unhelpful patterns of negative thinking.

Sometimes, life events, such as injury, illness, relationships, and mental and physical changes can shake our sexual confidence and mean we need to reshape our sexual ideas and adapt our sex lives to accommodate change. When we accept – as with the rest of our lives – that sex is in a constant state of flux, we can free our thinking and allow sex to take on a different meaning.

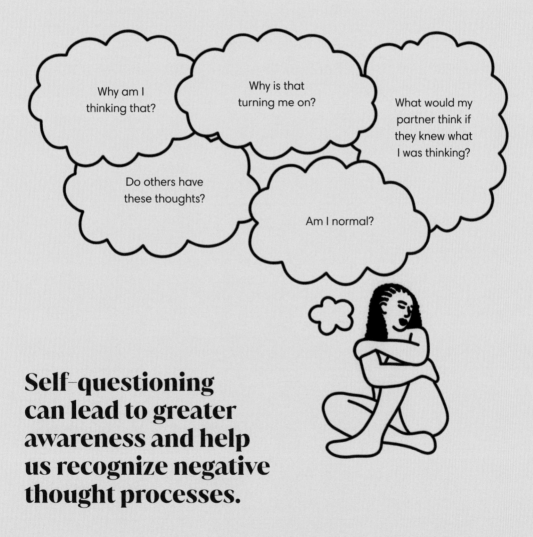

Self-questioning can lead to greater awareness and help us recognize negative thought processes.

Do we need to talk about sex?

When age-appropriate conversations about sex start at an early age and evolve during our lives, we normalize the topic, allowing us to communicate with partners and boost our sexual wellbeing.

When talking about sex is integrated into conversations across our lifetimes, this helps us appreciate the importance of communication and knowledge when it comes to sex. In some countries, such as the Netherlands, sex education is integrated into the curriculum from the age of four, teaching children in age-appropriate stages about consent, relationships, touch, love, and body parts. Conversely, when sex isn't discussed, this silence can indicate that the topic doesn't belong. As individuals, we may then internalize feelings of shame, leading to a sense of isolation, rather than recognize that this lack of conversation reflects a wider societal taboo.

Talking to partners

The way we talk about sex also matters. With verbal and non-verbal communication, indicators such as eye contact, body language, and tone of voice tell us how someone feels (see p.177). When these signals indicate discomfort, we struggle to have open, clear conversations. When it comes to partner-to-partner communication, many of us feel as though we're trying to hold a conversation in a language we haven't been taught. There's also an unspoken narrative that if we have to talk about sex, we must be doing something incorrectly – we should instinctively know how to have sex without needing to ask questions; or we can worry that a partner will feel criticized. Critically, not talking about sex is bad for our sex lives. All bodies and people are unique, and sex and pleasure are co-created between those

DON'T KNOW WHERE TO START?

Trying something new can feel hard. If you're unused to talking about sex with partners, try this simple exercise. Make a list together of sexual experiences. Separately, write "yes/no/maybe" for each one, then share your lists. This can be a non-pressured way to open up a dialogue and see where you might be similarly curious and/or express which practices you're not interested in.

involved, so each experience is different. When we feel unable to discuss sex, we may act based on inaccurate assumptions. We may also avoid opening up about what we enjoy or desire for fear of disappointing or upsetting a partner. This creates a cycle of carrying on with the same activities, even if these aren't working, rather than challenging the status quo. The longer this continues, the harder it is to speak up for fear a partner will wonder how long we've felt this way.

When we talk to partners about sex, this helps us explore our preferences and desires together, in turn leading to more pleasure (see below). We also deepen our sexual wellbeing and avoid feelings of shame that commonly arise when sex isn't working (see p.32).

The language we use

The words we use around sex infer meaning that can shape what we're doing sexually. For example, "foreplay" suggests there's an order, or plan, for how sex should happen, reinforcing the idea that intercourse is what matters. By changing our language and using the phrase "non-penetrative sex", we instantly reframe the narrative, opening up a world of possibilities inclusive of everyone, not just those having intercourse (see p.13).

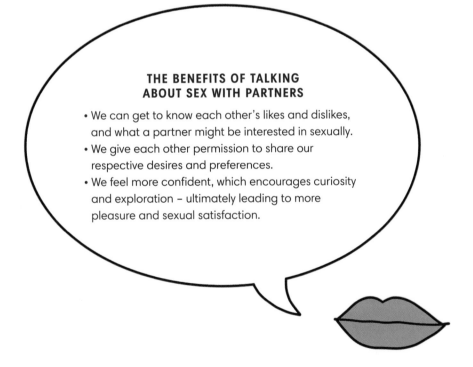

THE BENEFITS OF TALKING ABOUT SEX WITH PARTNERS

- We can get to know each other's likes and dislikes, and what a partner might be interested in sexually.
- We give each other permission to share our respective desires and preferences.
- We feel more confident, which encourages curiosity and exploration – ultimately leading to more pleasure and sexual satisfaction.

Does **solo sex** count?

Self-pleasure, solo sex, masturbation – whichever terminology we prefer – is a natural part of our sex lives, whether we're single or partnered and whatever our sexuality or gender identity.

For many of us, self-pleasure offers the chance to get to know ourselves in an environment free of expectation and/or the distraction of focusing on someone else's needs, or feeling that we're performing (see p.178). This may explain why people of all genders are more likely to orgasm when masturbating.

Despite this, a sense of shame is often felt around masturbation. This may come from cultural narratives and links back to historical urban myths, such as masturbating causing blindness. Such fearmongering was designed to control sexual desires by linking masturbation to fear and shame to keep sex within the realms of marriage.

Enjoying your solo playground

We can think about self-pleasure as being our own personal playground where we can do what we like for the sake of feeling good, and where there's no right or wrong.

There isn't a one-size-fits-all formula for masturbation. Some prefer practices that in no way resemble their partnered experiences; others like it to feel as close as possible to partnered sex. Self-touch can include different strokes, pressures, types of touch, and materials. Your preference may be to include erotic stimulation such as pornography, audio erotica, music, scent, sex toys, and lighting. You can use lubricant; masturbate in the shower or bath to enjoy the sensation of water; or you may enjoy positions that use your body weight to add sensation. Like partnered sex, solo sex is also down to our preferences at a particular time. Sometimes we may feel a desire to orgasm, while at other times, we can just enjoy sensations.

As with partnered sex, solo sex triggers the same feel-good neurochemicals, oxytocin and dopamine. It also helps us build our sexual sense of self and our relationship with our body so we can develop sexual self-confidence. In addition, it's the safest type of sexual experience we can have, carrying no risk of unwanted pregnancy or sexually transmitted infections.

Not for everyone

It's important to bear in mind that not everyone feels a desire to masturbate and that it's entirely down to personal preference. However, there's a difference between choosing not to masturbate because it's not your preference and avoiding it because of feelings of shame. One of the most critical parts of our sexual wellbeing is finding our own way and what we enjoy, rather than following what we feel we should be doing (see p.52).

UNRAVELLING MISCONCEPTIONS

A popular myth is that if we engage in solo sex when we're in a relationship, this means we're unsatisfied with our coupled sex. Actually, solo sex can be a great addition to our sex lives; by being curious, we bring self-knowledge and variety to partnered sex. Solo sex can also be an asset if one partner is unable to engage sexually, for instance during illness.

Some view solo sex as inferior to "real" sex. This links back to limiting cultural messages around intercourse being the sex that matters most, and completely devalues the experience of non-partnered people who can have satisfying, full sex lives. Solo sex is a valid and equal form of sexual expression.

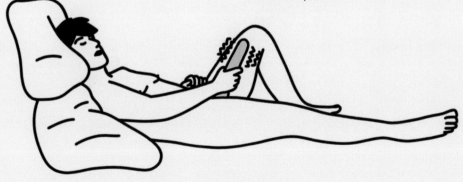

What does my partner like?

Entering into a sexual relationship with a partner involves a change in status. Learning to relate to each other sexually is key for satisfaction.

Enjoying sex with a partner, and understanding what turns them on, involves learning to communicate in a new way. We can pay attention to non-verbal and verbal cues; for example, they may encourage us with appreciative sounds or appear to get very turned on by having their ears kissed, so we continue to do this. We may read these cues correctly; however, we need to bear in mind that what someone shows us sexually in the moment may be shaped by what they consider socially acceptable, rather than reflecting their authentic desires. Being able to express our likes and dislikes openly is key.

Letting go of judgment

Misalignment of the meaning of sex between partners is a big predictor of the level of sexual satisfaction between them. Without good communication, we can clash over our understanding of the role of sex; for example, we may have different narratives around what's a "normal" amount of sex (see p.52). When we're able to discuss this, we can unpack how we feel and broaden the conversation to talk about what we like, what we're open to, and what we find exciting.

Truly exploring what turns a partner on therefore requires listening without judgment.

Part of this is being able to hear their likes and dislikes without personalizing what they say. Often when someone rejects a sexual act because it's not of interest to them, we take this as a personal rejection. If we reframe our thinking, making it clear we understand that this isn't the case, we create trust that allows us to explore and negotiate desires together.

The best time to talk

Ideally, talk to a partner about sexual preferences and desires at a neutral time, away from the bedroom. Being aware of the psychology of how we communicate can be helpful. For example, when we frame conversations positively, we can avoid a partner feeling criticized, which can make them shut down. Use "I" statements, such as, "I would love to know if there's anything you want us to try", which indicates you take ownership of your feelings.

If you've more than one partner, talk with each individually; or, if you're all having sex together, an honest group discussion can be helpful. When we change partners, we shouldn't assume that they'll enjoy the same things a previous person did. Being open-minded and not holding preconceived ideas (see p.20) about someone's desires can empower us to communicate clearly.

Sex can hold a unique meaning for each partner.

Clear communication about what you both like and dislike sexually has a cascade of benefits.

When we feel listened to, psychologically we feel accepted, which can increase our openness to sex.

We feel connected with our partner, which can enhance physical and emotional intimacy.

Physical pleasure can be maximized when we share desires successfully.

A positive loop of good communication and satisfying sex leads to repeated release of feel-good neurochemicals, such as oxytocin and endorphins.

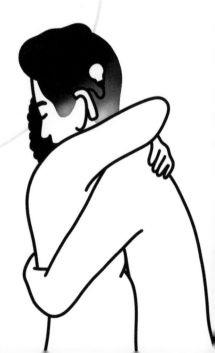

What's a non-monogamous relationship?

A consensual non-monogamous relationship describes the practice of having more than one sexual partner at a time. Making this work involves clear communication and consent.

There are no set rules for how non-monogamous relationships are structured, so they can look however we wish. Some relationships form by inviting others in; others involve partners having relationships or sex with partners outside of the relationship. With ethical non-monogamy, the importance is not what it looks like, but what's agreed, contracted, and communicated.

Won't we get jealous?

A common question is what's the difference between non-monogamy and cheating, and will this relationship model cause jealousy. Infidelity can happen in any relationship as cheating is about dishonesty. While jealousy can arise in a non-monogamous set-up, their consensual nature implies that communication is open and promotes discussions about feelings, so partners can unpack what's happening. Conversely, many in a non-monogamous set-up experience compersion – the opposite of jealousy, where they feel joy when a loved one experiences pleasure with another partner.

Opposite are examples of ethical non-monogamy terminology. Many people, though, don't feel the need to label relationship models, basing them instead on what feels good and works for their life, and adapting them as relations develop.

METAMOUR

This term describes your partner's partner, who you're not romantically or sexually involved with.

Open relationships are open to non-monogamous romantic and sexual possibilities, negotiated by all involved.

Monogamish is where relationships are monogamous most of the time, but sometimes partners agree sexual relationships outside of their set-up.

Kitchen table polyamory refers to the idea that all involved could sit around the kitchen table comfortably. It's not a fixed model but an approach to consensual non-monogamy. An opposing style is DADT – "don't ask, don't tell" – where the agreement is that partners don't know what the others are engaging in.

Throuple or triad is a triangular set-up where all have a romantic and sexual relationship with each other. **A quad** is where four people all date each other.

A closed V, like its shape, infers two partners share a romantic and/or sexual connection with a third partner, but not with each other.

Primary partner refers to a hierarchy in some non-monogamous relationships where the primary partner has the most significant relationship. Other relationships adopt an egalitarian structure, without hierarchy.

Swinging refers to those who are interested in new sexual connections but not necessarily romantic ones. Couples often swing together, with partner-swapping, swingers parties, or mixed groups being common ways of swinging.

DIFFERENT MODELS
These are just some examples of non-monogamous set-ups that operate within a pre-arranged agreement between all parties.

1 Couple or dyad

2 Triad

3 Quad

4 V or "Vee"

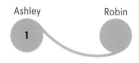

Ashley   Robin

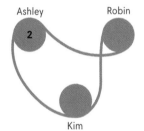

Ashley   Robin

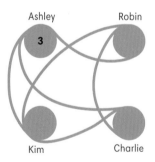

Kim

Ashley   Robin

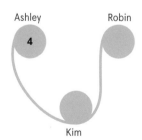

Kim   Charlie

Ashley   Robin

Kim

Why can sex feel shameful?

The origins of shame are often deep-rooted. We may not be consciously aware of them until we begin to question and examine why something is holding us back sexually.

Shame describes the emotion we feel when we think we've done something wrong. Unlike guilt, which focuses on specific actions, with shame we question our identity, feeling something is intrinsically wrong with us.

The way we learn about sex is often entwined with shame. We may pick up negative messages from caregivers or feel cultural expectations around sex. These may include having sex in certain contexts only, such as committed relationships; or ideas about genders behaving a certain way. Shame can therefore predate sexual exploration and unchallenged narratives become ingrained.

Other reasons for shame include worrying about lack of experience (see p.184); shame around fantasies; or shame of our bodies, for example, worrying about penis or labia size and symmetry. Shame is often reported by those seeking help for sexual problems, and shame and sexual challenges can exacerbate each other in a vicious cycle (see opposite).

The effect on sex

When it comes to sexual functioning, shame can feel so strong it creates a psychosomatic reaction (see opposite).

With our brains in "threat" response, rational thought in the prefrontal lobe shuts down and we enter fight-or-flight mode. The sympathetic nervous system is activated, increasing the heart rate and causing sweating, anxiety, and nausea. Emotionally, psychologically, and physically stressed, we can experience an urge to hide. This can cause psychological or physical discomfort, unease, or pain, interrupting desire and impacting sexual functioning.

Letting shame go

An antidote to shame is expressing ourselves, but often this makes us feel embarrassed and vulnerable. Despite modern-day society being saturated with sexual imagery, we can find it hard to normalize conversations around sex.

If we remove our experience of sex from social narratives, this can free our minds and how we think about sexual experiences. Being aware of our "self talk" – the positive or negative conscious and unconscious thoughts that form our inner dialogue – can help us think critically about where messages come from. Then we can offer ourselves compassion and find it easier to share problems.

THE SHAME CYCLE

A shame culture reinforces hard-to-break sexual thoughts, exacerbating self-criticism. Breaking away from the idea of goal-oriented sex can help us focus on what was good about an experience rather than what didn't work. Positive interventions can help break the negative loop.

Try not to overthink it. Social conditioning can make us quick to think we're failing if something isn't ideal.

Problems such as an inability to relax, reduced lubrication, or erection difficulties mean sex doesn't go to plan.

Self-criticism at this perceived failure leads to feelings of shame, reinforced by cultural, ingrained messages.

Feelings of shame increase, reinforcing sexual challenges.

Shame is one of the most common emotional responses to sex.

If we fail to communicate with partners, distracting thoughts mean there's an increased probability of sex not going to plan again.

Shame is interpreted as a threat, causing anxiety and a physiological fight-or-flight response.

In future, fear of failure adds stress, interrupting arousal and increasing the chance of failure. We can start to avoid sex.

Explaining how you feel to a partner now and/or maintaining contact, even if just hand-holding, can avoid feeling disconnected.

Breathing and mindful sex techniques (see p.180) that engage the parasympathetic nervous system can be calming.

Are sex and intimacy the same?

We often use the terms "sex" and "intimacy" interchangeably. However, they represent different parts of our relational experiences.

Intimacy is defined as a level of closeness between people. This can include physical and emotional intimacy, but doesn't require both for intimacy to exist. For example, we have close, intimate relationships with friends and family that aren't physical or sexual. Asexual people – who've little or no sexual attraction to others (see p.36) – can experience intimacy in this way. Intimacy is often described as having trust and the ability to be vulnerable, showing someone the true version of ourselves. Sex can clearly be part of intimacy and it's common to describe sex as intimate, but it isn't a vital component.

Our personal preferences

We're always cognitively engaged in sexual experiences, with sex involving a complex interaction of physical, cognitive, and psychological elements. However, despite this, we can have sex with a partner without intimacy or an emotional connection, which doesn't make it less valid.

Many find it easier to be sexually free with someone where there isn't a strong emotional connection. For some, the lack of emotion, or holding back emotionally, means there's less fear of rejection, which may be the case if trust is an issue. By safeguarding their emotions, even if subconsciously, they're able to let inhibitions go. Others find they feel higher levels of sexual satisfaction in relationships where there's a degree of familiarity and their partner knows their body – for them, intimacy is an important component of satisfying sex.

Mismatched expectations

Where both partner's views on the role of sex and intimacy align, there's little cause for distress. However, if there's a gap between desires, challenges can arise. For example, if we communicate attraction, affection, or love through sex but parters fail to reciprocate, we can make assumptions about how they feel, which can impact the satisfaction we feel. If we know we aren't seeking emotional intimacy, being upfront about this can

help manage expectations. Ultimately, if only one partner seeks intimacy, it's unlikely to provide the mutuality needed for both to be happy. While our ideas of what intimacy looks like can differ, understanding what it means to each partner can be helpful.

We can have sex without intimacy, and intimacy without sex.

Sex isn't a **priority,** is that okay?

There can be multiple reasons why someone may not desire sex. For some, this reflects their fundamental sexual orientation; for others, sex is deprioritized at certain times.

There's a huge variation in sexualities and sexual experiences, and the level of satisfaction, distress, or disinterest we experience around sex can decide whether it's something we desire. For some, it's useful to declare a lack of sexual interest as part of who they are; for others, variability and fluctuations in their sex lives reflect a specific phase or life stage. For example, we may notice that at certain times, for example when we're stressed, ill, or very preoccupied, that sex is deprioritized and desire drops.

Sexual definitions

Not feeling sexual attraction can be part of someone's sexual orientation, which is the case for asexual people. Asexuality is characterized by a lack of sexual attraction to others and an absent, or low, desire for sex. Asexuals may still have relationships, in the way that aromantics (see below) may still have sex, and people may be romantic asexuals, or both aromantic and asexual. Like everything in our sex lives, these labels exist on a spectrum (see opposite), dependent on each person's experience, preferences, and life events.

Aromantics have little or no romantic interest in others. Some also don't feel sexual attraction, while others do desire sexual connections. A common misconception about aromantics is that they're lonely and don't experience love, but aromantics can have fulfilling relationships in other ways; for example with families and friends, and, like many, they can have a love of places, hobbies, pets, and experiences.

THE ASEXUAL SPECTRUM

There are many misconceptions around asexual people, but, as with sexuality in general, asexuality describes a spectrum of preferences, related to individual variations of attraction, desire, and sexuality. Some feel more positive towards sex, others more neutral. Certain labels describe nuances within asexuality:

- gray-asexual describes someone who feels sexual attraction infrequently and/or not intensely.
- demisexuals need to form a close emotional bond before they can feel sexual attraction.

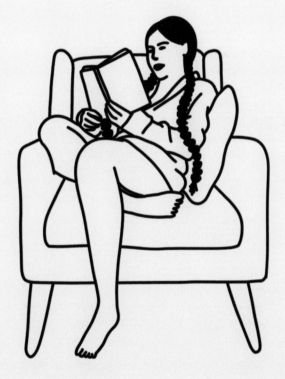

Can we get **better** at sex?

Much of the preoccupation around sex comes from the idea that there's a way to "do" it that can be learned and universally applied, making us good at sex in a measurable way.

Like any life skill, sex is a skill we develop. However, there isn't an official manual, nor does having more partners make us better at sex. Instead, sex is about discovery, learning by ourselves and with others while following overarching principles – treating others with respect; communicating; checking in with partners; and understanding our bodies and what we're happy to consent to.

Body knowledge – understanding the location and function of the parts of the body commonly associated with sex

(see p.69) – is one way we can develop sexual confidence. However, we can't know exactly what someone likes until we're in a sexual experience with them and learn the skill of communicating. Checking how partners feel, being confident asking questions, accepting differences, and exploring without judgment creates a positive framework in which we can grow our sexual skill set.

When our sexual experiences are positive in this way, confidence grows and we're more likely to be motivated to be open to future sexual experiences.

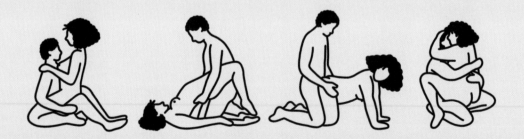

Sex is about respectful exploration.

What is
sexual wellbeing?

Our sexual wellness encompasses our emotional, physical, and psychological health. When we feel happy, confident, and comfortable generally, this can increase our sexual wellbeing.

Enhancing sexual wellbeing is about approaching sex in a multifaceted way – incorporating and integrating how we think about sex into how we feel about and relate to ourselves in general. When we do this, we're most likely to feel confident, happy, and comfortable sexually.

- **Open up your perspective** and consider what shapes your thinking about sex and whether you have a narrow view of what it's about. This can encourage curiosity, in turn activating the brain's reward system (see p.56) and helping us learn and discover new things about ourselves.
- **Think about your "self-talk"** – your inner dialogue with and about yourself. We're our own biggest critics, but when it comes to sex we need to be our own champions. Notice negative self-talk and push back, asking yourself, "Where's this thought coming from?" and then, "Is there another way to think about this?"

- **Identify barriers to sexual wellbeing** and give yourself permission to receive pleasure. For example, realizing we're constantly distracted can prompt us to think about how to focus more during sex. Or if sex is uncomfortable, is there something we can do differently, such as using lube (see p.86) that might help? We develop sexually once we make the decision to approach sex as a topic to be embraced, not ashamed of.
- **Connect with your body**. Our inner dialogue shapes how we see our bodies. Nurturing our body physically and celebrating what it can do, can help us gain sexual confidence in ourselves.
- **Accept yourself**. We all have different desires and preferences so avoid shaming yourself for who you are sexually. When we accept ourselves sexually, we're able to authentically be ourselves, which can boost our sex lives emotionally, psychologically, and physically.

What's sex about?

Sex is both simple and complex. As an experience, it's never isolated to the act alone; sex is shaped by the context of our lives and can shift as circumstances alter. Life changes as well as individual situations and preferences can affect how we experience desire, sometimes throwing up challenges. Understanding that how we define sex can be one of its biggest limitations can help us to pay attention to what's happening around us and how this impacts our sex lives. Looking at the role of our emotions, how our bodies feel pleasure, and the ways we can stimulate arousal can also help us to explore and embrace changes.

Does context change sex?

So much of our focus is on the physicality of sex. However, our brain is central to our experience of sex, and our motivation for having sex has the potential to transform the experience.

In their 2007 research paper, *Why Humans Have Sex*, psychologists David Buss and Cindy Meston questioned over 450 men and women on their motivations for having sex. The results uncovered 237 distinct reasons, ranging from emotional connection, to the desire to feel wanted, to experiencing orgasmic release, to relieving stress. Despite this huge variation in the reasons for having sex, there's a disproportionate focus on spontaneous desire (see p.130). In reality, our perspective and what's happening in our minds shape what we're experiencing.

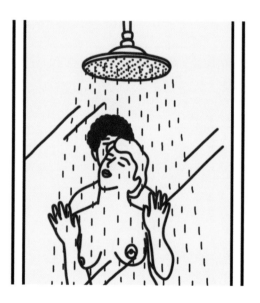

Sex isn't just about what we're doing, there is always an element of why.

Same scenario, different context

Context can affect our experience of sex in a variety of ways. For example, we may find we have time alone with a partner that offers an opportunity for physical closeness. If we feel relaxed and undistracted, we may take this chance to enjoy sex together. However, if in the same situation we're preoccupied by an external factor, such as a work worry, this can distract us and mean we aren't as open or responsive to each other.

Shifting reasons

What's happening in our lives and relationships can also change our context for sex and, in turn, impact the experience.

Often, when we first meet someone, sex is explorative and connecting. High levels of spontaneous desire at this time naturally lead to more frequent sex; this becomes a vehicle for showing interest in each other and, if wished, investing in building your connection.

Alternatively, if there has been a breach of trust in a relationship or a couple has drifted, sex may be a way to reconnect. The sex itself may or may not achieve this, but because of this motivation, partners may be more focused on and attentive to each other's responses as a way to decode their feelings.

Seeking an outcome

When trying to conceive, sex can become goal-orientated. At first, this can feel exciting, adding anticipation and acting as a positive motivator for sex. However, if sex becomes focused around ovulation, this can create pressure and reduce sex outside of this window. If conception is taking longer than anticipated, or if there's been previous pregnancy loss and/or struggles with fertility, anxiety can also creep in, and sex may move from being fun to more functional, impacting pleasure.

A conscious effort to focus on physical affection outside of your fertile window can help divert attention back to pleasure, rather than allowing sex to become purely outcome-orientated.

Can I ask a partner to wait for sex?

We often think of being ready for sex as a clearly defined moment. Setting aside embedded social narratives on when we should have sex can help you focus on your preferences.

Feeling ready for sex with someone is an individual choice that we should never feel pressured into, which goes hand in hand with consent (see p.20). Sex can be different things to each person. It follows therefore that a sexual experience is something that's ideally negotiated at an agreed pace, rather than based on a goal-achieving model of sex.

Putting it in context

Our sense of readiness for sex with someone, although influenced by them, is dependent on us. Deciding when to start a sexual relationship can also vary depending on the partner we're with and our context at that time. For example, if we've been emotionally hurt by an ex partner, we can feel more cautious with someone new. We can partly understand this when we think about how the brain processes pain. While emotional and physical pain aren't processed in exactly the same way, there's considerable overlap. With both, neural pathways in the insula and anterior cingulate cortex of the brain are activated. This helps explain why social rejection can feel so hurtful, and how a sense of caution may linger after emotional pain, as our brain fires off messages to stay away.

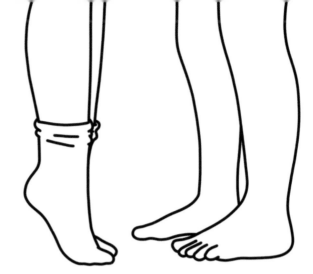

Physical needs

Physical changes can mean we need to assess when we're ready for sex. For instance, for some who've transitioned surgically, time can be needed to explore genital changes before having a sexual relationship. Or after childbirth, partners need to communicate when they're ready to resume sex. For those with disabilities, sex may need to be tailored to meet specific needs (see p.48); for instance, some basic prep, such as modifying positions or using aids, can help partners feel ready.

When the moment is right

While the timing of feeling ready for sex with someone new can be impacted by external factors and experiences, there isn't a set formula and our context can shift day to day. For example, if you begin to feel a connection and more emotionally confident around someone you're considering having sex with, then you may start to feel more open and ready for sex in the moment, rather than at a preconceived time. Equally, you can always stop a sexual encounter once it's started – an important part of consent is knowing that you can change your mind at any point.

How you both define sex and previous experiences are factors to consider. For instance, if penetration has been painful in the past (see p.120), exploring non-penetrative sexual activities initially can help build confidence.

There's no "right" time to start having sex with a partner.

Are we having enough sex?

The focus on how often we have sex has become a dominant measure for how successful we consider our sex lives. However, this offers limited information about sexual experiences.

Talking about the amount of sex we have is the most basic and obvious way to "measure" our sex lives. However, this makes no allowance for the quality of the sex we're having, which is the most important way to understand experiences. Thinking about how often we have sex is really only a consideration for couples working through issues such as discrepancies in desire (see p.136), or where thoughts of what's enough sex differ.

The best measure

Generally, regularity is a very sterile way to assess sex and poses the question of what we're measuring. If it's regularity of intercourse, does this mean that couples who don't have penetrative sex aren't having meaningful sex, or aren't having sex at all? Or that practices such as virtual sex don't count? How we shape what sex is can exclude many experiences that make sex meaningful and pleasurable.

The irony in worrying about quantity over quality is that the more enjoyable sex is, the more likely it is to lead to more sex. When we have great sex, we feel motivated to repeat this pleasurable experience and more likely to respond to a partner and lean into what's known as responsive desire (see p.130).

It's also important to acknowledge that for single people, how much sex they have relates to their number of partners. Often, this feeds into social narratives around an acceptable number of partners, rather than considering a person's subjective experience. Plus, for all, solo sex can be a constant source of pleasure, offering something different to partnered sex.

So what about the numbers?

While how much we have sex isn't a measure of a fulfilling sex life, some research shows that over the past two decades there's been a trend for couples to have less sex, with phrases such as "sex recession" or "sex drought" used. Other research suggests this may not be the case, and that studies focused on intercourse. There's no definitive answer, but one obvious possibility is that we may be prioritizing our smartphones and technology, which hijack our attention (see p.152). However, the link between sex and technology isn't wholly negative; many enjoy adapting their sex lives by including non-contact ways of being sexual, whether via phone sex, sexting, or virtual sex. Technology can also maintain sexual connection in long-distance relationships.

Talking to partners

If you do want to broach the topic with a partner of how much sex you're having, avoid positioning blame. Psychologically, using "I" statements shows ownership of our feelings. For example, "I feel so much closer to you when we've had sex recently" or, "Sometimes I worry about us when we're not having regular sex" or neutral statements such as, "We've been so busy, shall we spend time together this weekend?" This can avoid disagreements over sex and helps us understand each other's position. This type of communication can also act like a dictionary, translating our intimate desires.

Sex is a subjective experience that we can't measure objectively.

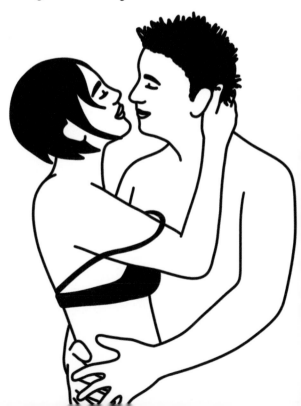

Will my disability affect sex?

The relationship between disability and sex is densely populated with myths, many of which come from an ableist position based on non-disabled assumptions.

A disability can be physical or mental, invisible or visible, and can impact all areas of a person's health and abilities. The word disabled is a huge umbrella term, within which each person has their own social contexts, which play a critical role in their lives generally and their sex lives. We can't assume what someone's sexual needs may be without talking to them about their preferences and how sex works for them.

Navigating sex around disability

While some share a type of disability, how it's experienced day to day and how it affects sex is dependent on individual circumstances. A disability may have been present at birth or acquired, sometimes from a progressive condition; in this case, we need to adapt our sex lives to navigate how our body is working and feeling. Being a disabled person living in an ableist society can also have an emotional and psychological impact on our experience of sex. From a practical point of view, we may experience a lack of privacy because of a need for carers to be present at times.

Unhelpful assumptions

One major obstacle for disabled people when it comes to sex is non-disabled people's assumptions. Many people believe that some disabled people don't desire to, or can't, have sex and disabled people are often socially desexualized. This ignores the reality that disabled people have the same desires and needs and enjoy intimate relationships. Some disabilities may mean that certain ways of being sexual aren't possible or need assistance or planning (see below), but this doesn't have to limit pleasure. As with everyone, sex can be expressed in many ways; what's most important is that it works for each individual.

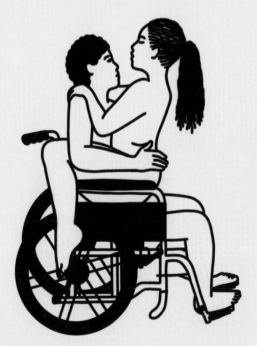

PHYSICAL AIDS

Historically, a lack of conversation around disability and sex meant that products weren't designed to help facilitate sex and pleasure for disabled people, leading to frustration at the barriers they faced.

Today, advances in design and greater awareness mean that products are available that help remove many obstacles to sex and pleasure a physically disabled person can encounter. For wheelchair users, sex swings or body hoists enable more partnered sex positions. There's also advances in sex toys, with pleasure products designed with specific disabilities in mind – for example, toys with adapted handles for those struggling with dexterity; sex toy mounts that make sex toys more accessible; and wedge cushions to make positions easier to get into.

Is it **just me** struggling with sex?

One of the primary concerns for those struggling with a sexual issue is the feeling that something with their sex life is broken and can't be fixed, and that they're the only one with a problem.

Experiencing a sexual problem, such as an erection issue (see p.122) or finding penetration painful (see p.120), can lead us to fear that our biological sexual functioning is broken and that this only affects us. However, studies show that sexual problems are common (see p.118) – it's thought that most people will encounter a sexual challenge at some point in their lives. Like every other area of our health and wellbeing, there's variability with sexual functioning, with good days and bad days. The fact that issues are commonplace indicates that problems are societal rather than individual, and it's the sexual culture surrounding us that's broken, not ourselves.

Despite this, the lack of awareness and education about how common sexual issues are means that when something goes wrong we feel a sense of personal failure. Sexual problems seem to exist in a vacuum – with information on how common issues are seldom discussed – which can lead us to feel shame around the topic (see p.32).

KNOCK-ON EFFECT

The figures below from the UK Natsal-3 study (see opposite) show how not dealing with sexual issues can impact our sex lives.

- ■ 13 per cent of women who'd had sex in the past year avoided sex at times because of sexual difficulties.
- ■ 11 per cent of men who'd had sex in the past year avoided sex at times because of sexual difficulties.

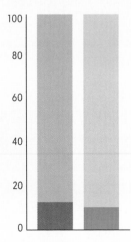

Failing to seek help

We experience feeling sexually broken differently to being physically broken. When ill or injured, others often notice and we're likely to seek help. The sense of shame we can feel around sexual issues can make it harder to reach out. Society has moved forwards, normalizing conversations around sex more, but sexual health and wellbeing still isn't prioritized; as a result, we continue to suffer gaps in our sexual understanding (see pp.168–189), exacerbating problems.

There's evidence that, the older we are, the less we worry about sexual problems. The UK Natsal-3 (National Survey of Sexual Attitudes and Lifestyles) study showed that while sexual problems tend to increase with age, the distress we report decreases. This suggests that the expectation of a problem is normalized the older we get, so we feel more equipped psychologically to deal with it. Again, this indicates how social influences can play a key role in how we understand ourselves.

Common side effects of struggling with sex are feelings of shame and isolation.

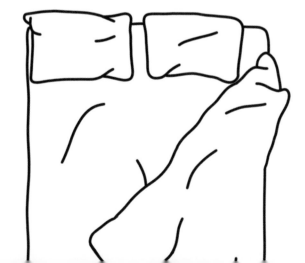

Is my sex life normal?

When it comes to sex, we're preoccupied with what's "normal". What's a normal amount of sex? How long should it last? What's the right range of sexual activities and desires?

To be accepted – to fit in – is a basic human instinct. In evolutionary terms, being part of a cooperative social group meant survival. Belonging is a powerful pull and we see being normal as avoiding the risk of social rejection. This fear is real as social rejection is thought to impact our emotional, cognitive, and physical health.

In terms of sex, we hold strong ideas about what's normal. Socially, we live in a heteronormative society – where heterosexuality is prioritized. Many of us fear that not being seen as normal says something intrinsic about us. The desire to be normal can also influence how we feel about our bodies and genitals and our ability to be comfortable showing another person our body.

The concept of "should sex"

Driven by the fear of rejection, we can behave in ways that are aligned more with how we think we *should* behave sexually, rather than how we authentically wish to be. This helps explain why so many struggle with sex (see p.178) and why those who have sex that aligns with their desires – rather than trying to fit into what they believe is expected – often report satisfying sex lives.

Our sex lives are frequently guided and shaped by a sexual "script" that we learn via socialization and culture. These norms dictate what's acceptable or appropriate and act as a conscious and unconscious guide for how we should think, feel, and act sexually. Embedded in us is the idea that going off-script will have negative

Like every aspect of our lives, our sex lives are full of nuance, reflecting our unique circumstances.

consequences; we therefore use this blueprint as a reference point to measure ourselves against. One of the most frequently asked questions when it comes to sexual worries is, "Am I normal?"

Questioning sexual scripts

Many of us never explicitly consider our sexual scripts. A useful exercise is to note the unspoken rules, or framework, you manage your sex life by. For example, consider what you think sex should involve. Do you think sex for you should be with a certain type of person, or make you feel a certain way? What defines good and bad sex? You may also have thoughts about how long you think sex should last; whether you should both orgasm; that you should know what a partner likes without asking; and that you should know what you're doing. Once you've done this, go back and question, "Why do I think that?"; "Where's that thought from?"; and "Is that belief working for me?"

Addressing our scripts lets us rewrite our sexual narratives. For instance, if you're experiencing erection issues or painful sex, are you focusing too much on getting sex right rather than on whether it's pleasurable? Or does your sexual script mean sticking to a label that may be stopping you trying something you desire (see p.186)? When it comes to sex, thinking about what's normal is counterintuitive and holds us back. Just as there are variations with other aspects of our lives, there's no "normal" for our sex lives.

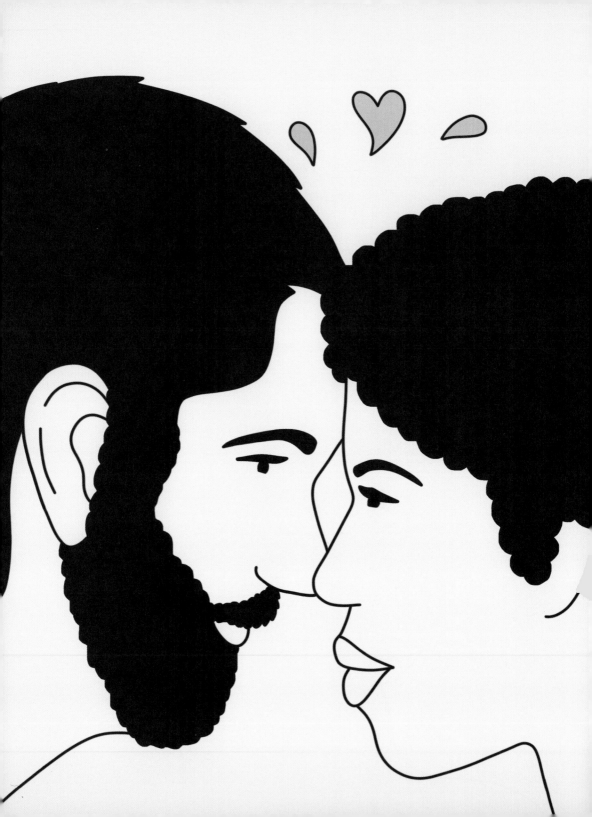

Is feeling emotionally vulnerable after sex normal?

Sex can be an exposing and vulnerable experience, particularly as we use it as a way to connect physically, emotionally, and psychologically.

We're biochemically primed to connect via sex as the release of oxytocin and endorphins plays a critical role in bonding. Even with casual hook-up sex, we activate and release neurochemicals that prime us to feel momentarily closer to someone.

Some find sex so intense that they cry. There's no exact science for this, but theories include tears being a natural response to intensity; hormone fluctuations in sex triggering tears; or, for some, sex having powerful positive or negative connotations. Studies show that tears shed emotionally have a higher number of stress hormones than lubricating tears or those triggered by irritants.

Rethinking vulnerability

Many of us are taught that vulnerability is a weakness, but numerous experts have reframed it as a strength that allows for more compassion, less judgment, and deeper intimacy.

Intimacy is deepened when we show another person who we authentically are, and many of these connecting moments can happen during sex, with eye contact, sensual touch, and pleasure. When we let ourselves go sexually this can be intimate and primal, with orgasm taking us into an altered state. When we're comfortable enough to let go sexually, we can focus on pleasure without holding back, rather than try to manage how others see us. Allowing ourselves to lose control with someone can be deeply connecting as the boundaries between us blur temporarily.

POSTCOITAL DYSPHORIA (PCD)

PCD can occur after consensual, satisfying sex. It's characterized by post-coital feelings of sadness, irritability, or tearfulness. While more research is needed, a 2015 paper found 46 per cent of women had experienced PCD at least once, and a 2019 study found it had affected 41 per cent of men.

What is
pleasure?

Pleasure is one of life's biggest motivators. While pleasure can be subjective – some derive it from thrill-seeking pursuits, others from simple activities – we all like things that make us feel good.

We learn what gives us pleasure through a combination of genetics, biology, learning, and experience, and how we experience pleasure is shaped by social, cultural, and environmental factors.

As humans, our cognition – how we think – plays a part in how we engage with pleasure as we sometimes have to make goal-directed decisions, weighing up the potential value or consequences of actions. This process plays a big part in risk-taking and building habits; it's why we sometimes act on impulse, making decisions motivated by immediate reward rather than long-term consequences. A person described as hedonistic is considered a pleasure-seeker, orienting their life towards the pursuit of pleasure and feeling good above other experiences. In the context of sex, we're motivated to have sex when we feel it's rewarded by pleasure.

The role of dopamine

The neurochemical dopamine plays a critical role in pleasure. It's released in anticipation of a pleasurable experience. The brain's dopamine pathways – mesolimbic and mesocortical – are activated when we experience something rewarding such as sex (see opposite). This feel-good neurotransmitter therefore plays a role in reinforcement behaviours as we're encouraged and motivated to go back for more.

Intense sensations

Physically, the areas of the body with the highest density of nerve endings are linked to the highest intensity of pleasure and pain (see p.88). Our brain processes these sensations, communicating via the nervous system as to what feels good or not. This is tempered by our social environment, or how we feel about what we're doing. So for some, an activity might feel good physically, but emotionally is negative. When what feels good is aligned physically and psychologically, this can push pleasure to new heights.

In practices such as BDSM (see p.146), pain and pleasure co-exist. This is because endorphins are released with pain, creating sensations of heightened intensity.

PLEASURE PATHWAYS

Dopamine is made in the ventral tegmental area (VTA) of the midbrain. During rewarding experiences, it's activated, then travels to different parts of the brain via the dopamine pathways.

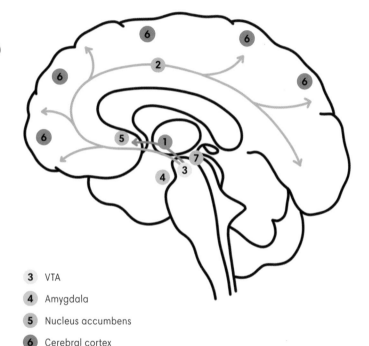

1 **Mesolimbic pathway**
This sends dopamine from the VTA to the nucleus accumbens. It links to the hippocampus and amygdala, attributing feelings and memory to pleasurable events such as sex.

2 **Mesocortical pathway**
This takes dopamine from the VTA to the cerebral cortex, bringing our consciousness to the experience of pleasure.

3 VTA

4 Amygdala

5 Nucleus accumbens

6 Cerebral cortex

7 Hippocampus

The chemical reward of dopamine motivates us to repeat pleasurable experiences.

What about sex toys?

Sex toys can introduce new sensations, experiences, and ways of engaging in sexual play during solo and partnered sex. Knowing what's on offer can help you choose the best toy for you.

Sex toys are designed for pleasure. Some worry that using one suggests their sex life is lacking or they're unhappy with a partner. In fact, they can offer new insights into pleasure, knowledge that can be taken into partnered activities. For those who struggle to orgasm, intense stimulation from a sex toy can focus attention and be a very useful tool.

Choosing and using sex toys

- **Some toys are dual purpose**, for example, stimulating the G spot (see p.84) and clitoris together; others, such as prostate massagers, focus on one area. Dildos are often phallus-shaped; strap-on ones come with a harness so they can be used like a penis. Vibrators add pleasure by creating movement through vibrations or oscillations; they can be used all over the body, building pleasure and sensation. Toys with suction cups can be attached to solid surfaces, such as a shower wall, allowing hands-free fun. There are also toys designed for humping and grinding rather than penetration, for those who enjoy the sensation of pushing against something.

- **Some toys are designed for specific users**, for instance, for those with physical disabilities or hand limitations. There are also products for trans bodies that take into account changes in genital size and sensation.

- **Choose toys made of body-safe materials** that are phthalate-free. Non-porous materials such as silicone are safest as porous ones can harbour infection-causing bacteria. Toys can also be made of stainless steel and borosilicate glass, which help conduct temperature changes if wished.

- **For anal play**, choose toys with a flared base to prevent strong anal muscles sucking a toy into the anal cavity (see p.87).

- **Clean toys after each use** to stop bacterial build up and STI transmission. If you've used a toy for anal play and want to use it elsewhere, clean it first; or, if you used a condom, change this to avoid transferring bacteria from the anus.

- **Use water-based lube** with toys; silicone- or oil-based ones can damage materials, making toys unsafe.

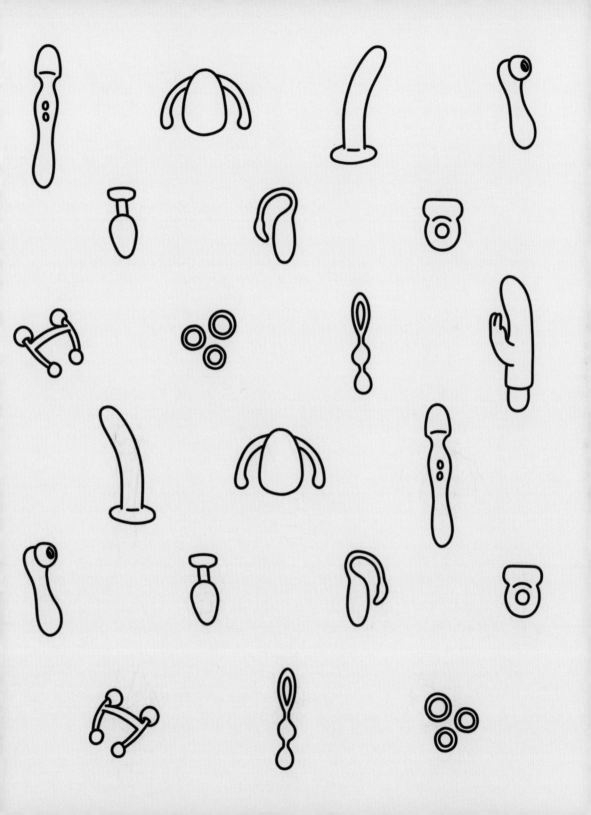

What about **porn?**

Many find porn pleasurable, but being aware that some porn can impact our ideas about sex is also important.

Porn is enjoyed by millions, incorporated into both partnered and solo sexual experiences. There's a huge diversity of pornography. For some, seeing their particular kink, fetish, or sexuality represented in a way that isn't often seen in mainstream media can feel affirming, breaking away from a set perception of pleasure and sex.

Looking at the challenges

While pornography has existed throughout history, from explicit depictions in cave drawings to early erotic photography, the invention of the internet and smartphones heralded an explosion in widely accessible free porn. This has seen many young people turn to porn for answers to sexual questions. However, it's important to recognize there's a difference between pornography and real-world sex and that porn is designed to arouse, not educate. For those who've had early and continued exposure to pornographic content, it can be harder not to blur the lines between porn and reality.

A new wave of ethical pornographers are encouraging "porn literacy". This aims to increase awareness of the exploitative and often violent porn many consume and offer ethical alternatives. Erika Lust, a Swedish erotic film director, creates porn that promotes equal pleasure for all (see opposite). While Cindy Gallop, founder of MakeLoveNotPorn, has set up the world's first user-generated and human-curated "social sex" platform; this breaks away from the choreographed, unrealistic depictions of sex and pleasure in much mainstream porn, offering a real-world representation of the sex people have.

The world of erotica

While visual pornography is most arousing for some, others find visual images distracting. In this case, written and audio erotica/porn allows someone to create their own imagery and use their imagination. They can construct a fantasy that's perfectly tailored to them, reflecting what they find most desirable and arousing.

WHAT MAKES PORN ETHICAL?

Porn director and producer Erika Lust cites eight key principles for ethical porn:

- **Pleasure is equal**; women are active, not passive, participants, with their own needs.
- **Diversity is key**. People are represented equally and performers aren't reduced to factors such as body shape or ethnicity.
- **Fair pay** is ensured for all involved.
- **Transparency** is a given. Each person is credited as part of the team.
- **A safe-sex environment** is promoted; all performers have up-to-date STI checks and are clear on the protection they're using.
- **There are no surprises** for performers. Each part of a film is agreed in advance.
- **There are high workers' standards**, with sufficient breaks, refreshment, and a welcoming atmosphere.
- **Fair commissions** are ensured for each director and studio.

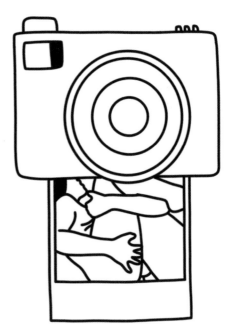

How do we avoid a sex rut?

The difference between being in a sexual routine and a sex rut is the level of satisfaction or dissatisfaction you feel.

A rut is associated with feeling stuck, as though you can't move on. Feeling that your sex life is in a rut can happen when you struggle to break away from ingrained ideas about how we have sex – for example, expecting sex to be linear, starting with "foreplay" and ending in intercourse (see p.92). One or both partners can fail to challenge set sexual scripts. Often, our general awkwardness around sex holds us back so we can avoid suggesting trying something different, compounding the sense of being stuck. While getting into a sex rut is not at all uncommon, what's important is how we deal with it once we find ourselves there.

BREAKING OUT OF A RUT

The steps below offer a framework for working with a partner to bring about changes to your sex life.

Step 1
Consciously address the situation. Starting the conversation about changing what's not working for you can be one of the hardest things to do. Focus on your sexual relationship and feelings and avoid assigning blame, which can lead to conflict.

Step 2
Tune into your motivation for change. Identify sexual patterns and beliefs that you want to address to make bringing about change feel manageable.

Recognizing habitual behaviour

A lack of curiosity can limit our capacity for learning; in relationships, one of the biggest traps is thinking that we know exactly what a partner likes. Sexual habits can easily form as repeated behaviour becomes automatic. Habitual behaviour starts when our brain is motivated to chase the feel-good high we get from dopamine during sex (see p.56), building a connection between a previous action and pleasure. But as we get used to something, we fail to respond as much, known as habituation. This is helpful when it stops us reacting unnecessarily to repeated stimuli, such as background noise, but unhelpful for sex.

We need to address habituation consciously in our sex lives to be able to bring about change. Small shifts – such as those suggested in step three below – help us to grow in confidence sexually and to explore more, leading us to discover new things about a partner and ourselves.

When we break away from a linear model, instantly we have more options and the freedom to do what we wish in no particular order. In terms of neurochemistry, the dopamine boost we get from new pleasures encourages us to try something again, building desire so we're likely to have more sex that's more fulfilling.

Step 3
Take small steps. Trying to overhaul your entire sex life can feel daunting; success is most likely with gradual, agreed changes. Communicate unambiguously and positively. For instance, "There's a position I'd like to try, would you be up for something new?"; or, "Shall we change the order of how we do things?" Alternatively, dim the lights rather than turn them off, start with clothes on or off, or try changing who initiates sex.

Step 4
If you're met by your partner's resistance, ask them what they think you could try that could work for you both. It's important you feel heard and understood, but also that you both have a chance to say no to trying something new. Accept that it's rare to be perfectly aligned in our sexual preferences.

Can fantasies enhance sex?

Our imagination and curiosity is part of what makes us human. Allowing our minds to wander when it comes to sex is perfectly natural and can even have positive outcomes.

According to research by US psychologist Dr Justin Lehmiller, 97 per cent of us have sexual fantasies, and for many, fantasies are frequent. Often, though, we unnecessarily shame ourselves for fantasizing, reinforcing the connection between sex and shame, which can be detrimental to our sex lives (see p.32).

A way to enhance sex

When embraced, fantasies can boost our sex lives by introducing a new element without physically doing anything new, releasing dopamine to trigger the brain's reward pathways (see p.56). We can also use fantasies as a cue to draw our mind to sex – getting us in the mood or building desire once we're having sex and, in turn, evoking an arousal response (see p.93).

The fact that we have fantasies isn't inherently the sign of a problem within a relationship, unless we're aware of being dissatisfied. We tend to have a romanticized view that when we're with a romantic or sexual partner, they should meet our every need, so fantasizing indicates that there's something lacking. Interestingly, Lehmiller's research found that 90 per cent of people say they've fantasized about their current partner before. It also showed that, generally, sharing fantasies brought couples closer and increased intimacy. When partners don't feature, this doesn't mean that we're interested in acting out our fantasy in real life, as desire and fantasy, while overlapping, are different concepts. Being curious is entirely natural as our brains constantly engage with the world around us; for many, fantasies are simply a safe way to explore in our minds without involving anyone else.

Do fantasies have meaning?

Often if we try to understand the meaning of fantasies, we give them too much attention. This isn't always helpful because when it comes to sexual fantasies, we're often self-critical. While not conclusive, one study using brain imaging scans estimated that we have more than 6,000 thoughts a day. With that in mind, it's probably less important to focus on the content of thoughts and more how we treat them.

TOP FANTASIES

Lehmiller's survey on 4,175 men and women aged 18-87, published in his 2018 book *Tell Me What You Want*, included a variety of genders and sexualities. Across all groups, certain fantasies were particularly popular (see right). Other popular themes involved romance and intimacy and non-monogamy and partner-sharing.

Sometimes fantasies relate to things we've previously enjoyed, sexually or otherwise; the positive connection between that act, place, or person is established, making it a reliable memory to revisit and enjoy. A sense of familiarity can play a key role in fantasies if the repetition of familiar scenarios allows us to relax and feel aroused. We can have fantasies about people we feel strongly about, including those that we intensely dislike, or we can fantasize about things detached from our reality, but our fantasies don't have to make sense. Sometimes fantasies might be telling us about our needs, but they can also simply be about our capacity for imagination.

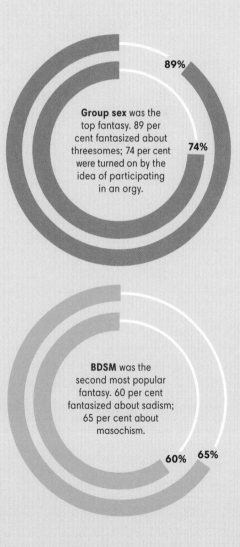

89%

Group sex was the top fantasy. 89 per cent fantasized about threesomes; 74 per cent were turned on by the idea of participating in an orgy.

74%

BDSM was the second most popular fantasy. 60 per cent fantasized about sadism; 65 per cent about masochism.

60% **65%**

Body knowledge

Understanding our sexual bodies – using the correct terminology for our sexual anatomy and being aware of how our bodies function when we have sex – has hugely positive implications for our sexual health and wellbeing. In this chapter, become knowledgeable about your sexual body: discover what's going on in your brain and body during arousal and at the peak of pleasure; get clued up on how our sex hormones impact sex; and learn how different sexual positions can contribute to pleasure. Being aware of what's happening during sex will also help you recognize when something isn't working sexually and give you the confidence to seek timely advice.

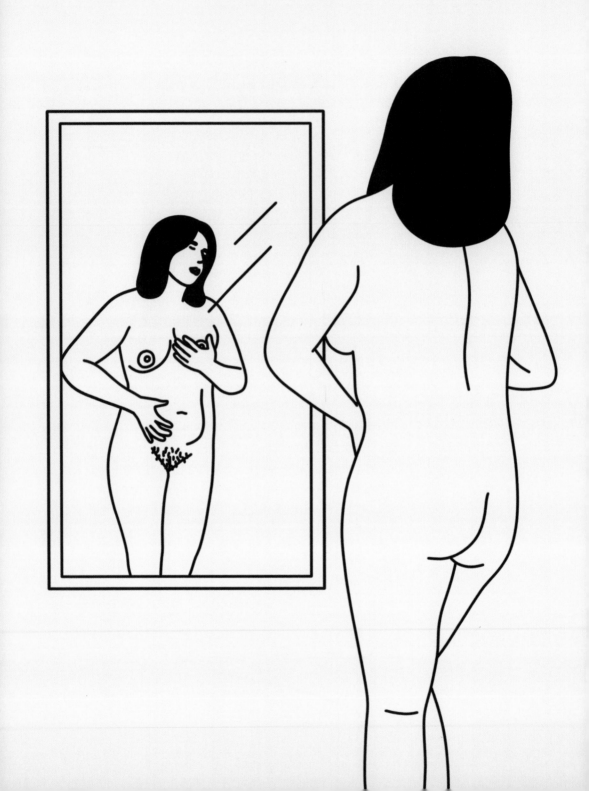

Why does knowing my body help my sex life?

Our level of awareness about our own bodies impacts so many parts of our lives. It may seem a given that as we exist daily in our bodies we know them instinctually, but often this isn't the case.

Our body knowledge affects many aspects of our sex lives, often without us realizing. When we're aware of how our bodies work, this helps us to explore what's pleasurable; understand our preferences and when we feel we wish to give or withhold consent; and enhances our body confidence – all building blocks for sexual confidence. For example, when we engage with self-exploration, we can discover what we like sensually and sexually and can tell a partner more confidently what feels good. Or, if our bodies change – during illness, injury, childbirth, or gender-affirming hormonal or surgical treatment – taking time to explore these changes helps us to become reacquainted with ourselves.

Being well informed

Good body knowledge also enhances our health literacy – our ability to understand health information. This in turn allows us to take charge of our own sexual health and wellbeing and to make informed choices around important areas such as how to protect ourselves against sexually transmitted infections and avoid unwanted pregnancies. Despite this, research consistently shows that our body knowledge is poor. In one US poll of 2,000 women, nearly one in four were unable to identify the vagina correctly and 46 per cent couldn't locate the cervix. Elsewhere, myths persist around issues such as erectile dysfunction and painful sex (see p.95 and p.120). This likely reflects how the sex education we receive is often lacking. In a 2021 UK Sex Education Forum survey of over 1,000 young people, only around 35 per cent rated their school's sex ed programme as good or very good. Many of us use incorrect terminology or slang for parts of our genitals, and evidence suggests that uptake for medical advice about our genitals or sexual issues is often delayed as people feel ashamed or embarrassed. When it comes to our genitals, so often we simply aren't encouraged to learn about ourselves – to explore and be curious.

Understanding the barriers that can stop us getting to know ourselves helps us rebuild our relationship with our bodies and fully enjoy the pleasure they can offer.

Am I normal down there?

Variety in our bodies is usual, however, when it comes to our genitals, we're often curious to know whether our own look "normal". In fact, no penis or vulva is exactly the same.

Any part of our bodies can be sexual, but the parts most commonly associated with sex are our genitals. The limited representations we see of these – often from unrealistic, edited sources in the online world and pornography – can create anxiety about how we measure up.

Diversity in our genitals is expected, with a huge variety in skin colour, shape, and size. Bear in mind, too, that during puberty the shape of our external genitalia is still evolving.

- No two vulvas (see p.72) look the same. The folds of skin here – the labia – come in a wide range of lengths and thicknesses, and the clitoris (see p.76) may be visible or hidden under a hood. Despite this, many people feel self-conscious and insecure about the appearance of their vulva. One of the fastest-growing cosmetic surgery procedures is labiaplasty, which modifies the appearance of the labia minora, often to align with a perceived vulval "norm".
- Penises (see p.78) have varying lengths, thicknesses, and shapes. In a circumcised penis, the foreskin has been removed.

- Our genitals are often a darker skin tone than other parts of the body as they have a higher number of melanin-containing pigment cells, which are sensitive to the effects of oestrogen and testosterone. In addition, during arousal, increased blood flow to the genitals can make them appear temporarily darker or take on a purplish hue.
- Pubic hair varies widely in texture, amount, and colour.
- For those medically transitioning with hormone treatment or surgery (see p.82), the genitals and their function will change as they go through this process.
- Some are born with a natural variation of sex characteristics that don't fit typical binary notions of male or female, referred to as being intersex. For some, this may be discovered later, with secondary sexual development.

The most important thing is to identify your own normal, which will allow you to recognize any changes that occur, understand these, and seek further advice when needed.

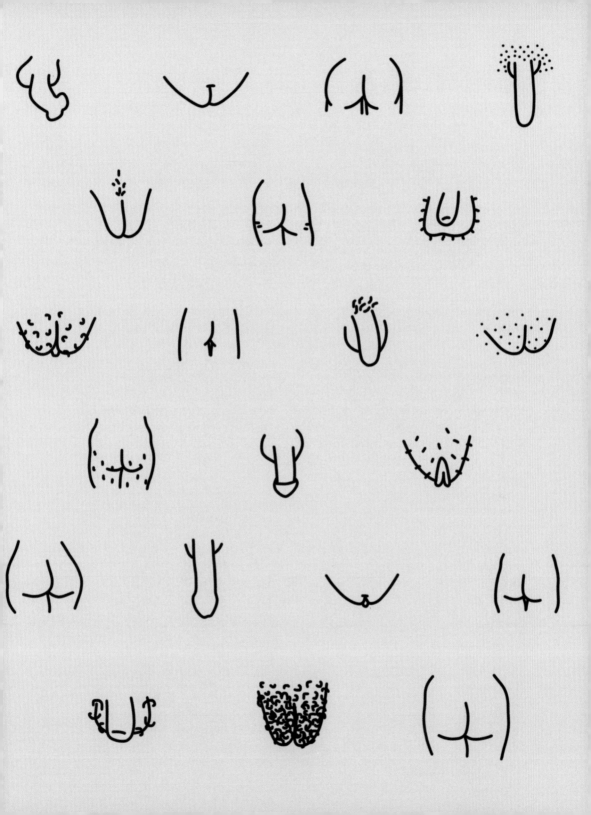

Vagina or vulva?

Our terminology around the vulva and the internal vagina is often confused and misused. Understanding the arrangement of these genitals clarifies their structure and function.

Colloquially, people often use the word vagina to describe a vulva. This is problematic as it erases a critical part of the sexuality of those with a vulva, reducing function to being reproductive rather than pleasure-based. It puts the emphasis on the part of the anatomy – the vagina – most focused on penetration, sidelining the clitoris and rest of the vulva, which are the parts that most people report receiving sexual pleasure from. It also prevents people with a vulva from clearly describing and communicating about their body, whether for pleasure or health. As the entirety of these genitalia isn't easily visible – especially as the vagina is an internal canal – using a hand mirror to explore your genitals is the best way to get familiar with them and be comfortable with your normal.

VULVA
This is the umbrella term for all the external parts of these genitals. It includes the vaginal opening but not the vaginal canal.

1. Vaginal opening
2. Mons pubis
3. Labia minora
4. Labia majora
5. Glans clitoris
6. Clitoral hood
7. Urethral opening

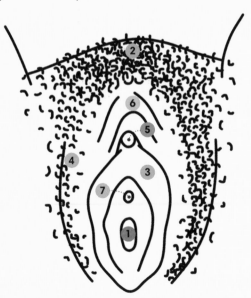

The vulva

This is the outer part of the genitals – everything you can see externally. It comprises the vaginal and urethral openings, the labia minora, labia majora, mons pubis, and glans clitoris.

- **The vaginal opening**, sometimes called the introitus, gives access to the inner vagina (see right). This area is sensitive to stimulation so can play a part in sexual pleasure. Between the vaginal opening and anus is the perineum.
- **The mons pubis** is the mound of fatty tissue, naturally covered in pubic hair, that lies over the pubic bone and extends to the clitoral hood. It provides cushioning during intercourse and is sensitive to touch itself so can build up anticipatory pleasure.
- **The labia minora** – the inner lips – sit next to the labia majora (see opposite and right). They're thinner and more sensitive than the labia majora and can be longer and more folded. Their length and appearance varies hugely and they're usually not identical or symmetrical - in sexology, both sets of labia are described as sisters, not twins. The labia minora are covered with a mucus membrane. When aroused, increased blood flow to this area can cause them to change colour and become thicker and more sensitive, making touch to the area highly pleasurable.

- **The labia majora** – outer lips – are thicker, cushioned skin folds. The skin is the same as the rest of the body so pubic hair can grow here. Also responsive to touch, the area protects more delicate parts of the vulva such as the labia minora and vaginal entrance.
- **The glans clitoris** – the external clitoral nub – is an area of spongy tissue towards the front of the vulva by the mons pubis. It swells when aroused and is the centre of sexual pleasure for most people with a clitoris (see p.76).
- **The urethral opening** is found in the vulva vestibule – the smooth area around the urethral and vaginal openings. It's located between the clitoris and the vaginal entrance. This opening transports urine out of the body. As it's close to the vagina, it's advisable to urinate after sex to flush out any bacteria that could cause a urinary tract infection.

The vaginal canal

The muscular internal canal of the vagina (see p.74) connects the opening of the vagina to the cervix – the neck of the womb, or uterus.

What happens to the vagina during sex?

The vagina is described as a potential space as it's highly elastic and easily expandable when it needs to be – for example during penetration, when using a tampon, or in childbirth.

Several processes take place in the vagina during sex that help to prepare it for penetration and increase sexual pleasure. When aroused, the vagina actually changes its size in a process called "tenting" (see opposite), whereby the body draws the uterus upwards to create more length in the vaginal canal for comfortable penetration. Figures vary, but some estimate that the vagina increases from 7–8cm (2¾–3¼in) to 11–12cm (4–4¾in). The vaginal walls are also textured – lined with transverse ridges called rugae. These play an important part in allowing the vagina to expand during penetration and childbirth. Trans women who've had a vaginoplasty procedure (see p.83) to form a neovagina sometimes experience vaginal restriction so may be advised to use vaginal dilators (see p.120)

post-surgery to stretch the vaginal canal and help keep it open.

The vagina is also self-lubricating, with several sources of lubrication. Vaginal discharge, produced by the vagina and cervix, occurs throughout the menstrual cycle and is completely normal; its role is to keep the vagina protected, clean, and moist. Cervical fluid changes in texture and viscosity throughout a cycle, with increased fluid around the time of ovulation helping to lubricate the vagina during sex. Reflex responses to arousal create extra lubrication. The vaginal walls are covered with a moist mucus membrane. When we're aroused, blood flow to the walls increases, causing them to swell and fluid to pass through them, in turn increasing sensitivity. In addition, either side of the vaginal opening, small pea-like

The amount of wetness produced during arousal is outside of our conscious control.

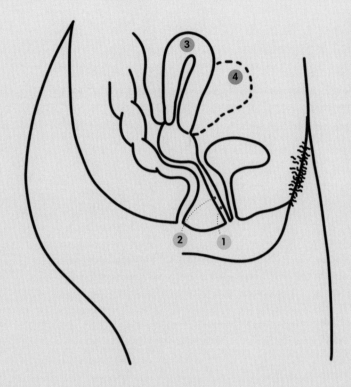

THE TENTING PROCESS
During arousal, the uterus lifts up, allowing the vagina to lengthen by several centimetres to increase comfort during penetration.

1 Vagina

2 Rugae – vaginal ridges

3 Uterus – during arousal

4 Uterus – normal state outside of arousal

structures called Bartholin's glands secrete fluid during arousal, while the Skene's glands, either side of the urethra, secrete mucus-containing fluids during sex to help lubrication. These lubricating processes reduce friction and the risk of damage to the vaginal walls during penetration and help ensure that intercourse is comfortable and pleasurable. For trans women who've had surgery to construct a vagina, additional lubrication is recommended to ensure sex is comfortable.

A sensitive area

While the vagina plays a key role in intercourse and penetrative sex – and for those having sex with the purpose of trying to conceive – it can also be a source of pleasure without penetration. Most of its nerve endings are in the lowest third, closest to the entrance, and so stimulation of this area can provide plenty of pleasure and enjoyment as part of sexual play without full penetration.

What does the clitoris do?

Our understanding of the full structure and function of the clitoris is fairly recent. The arrival of MRI scans dramatically increased our knowledge around this pleasure-giving organ.

Direct stimulation of the clitoris is the most commonly reported way for people with a vulva to reach orgasm, with one study citing that 81.6 per cent need additional clitoral stimulation during intercourse to climax. Packed with nerve endings, the only known function of the clitoris is for pleasure. However, this part of the anatomy is often left out of mainstream sex education, where the primary focus is on intercourse – as recently as the 1948 edition of Gray's Anatomy, the clitoris was excluded. The result is that the sexual pleasure of people with a vulva is effectively de-prioritized, helping to explain statistics such as those revealed in the gap between the orgasm rates in people with a vulva compared to those with a penis in heterosexual partnered sex (see p.170).

What we can see

The tip of the clitoris – the external part we can stimulate directly – is called the glans. This is protected by the clitoral hood, which sometimes obscures the external clitoris from view. You can manually push the hood up slightly towards your body to reveal more of the clitoris glans during solo or partnered play. As with the penis, the most sensitive area of the clitoris is the glans – the part with the greatest density of nerve endings.

More than meets the eye

The most famous study on the clitoris was carried out by Australian urologist Helen O'Connell. Working mainly with MRI scans, she revealed the full anatomy of the clitoris for the very first time in 2005, creating a ground-breaking 3-D model. Far from being just a pea-sized spot on the vulva, the clitoris is in fact a mostly subterranean organ – often described as being like an iceberg. Around 90 per cent of its entire structure sits below the surface, extending into the pelvis and down either side of the vagina.

The internal body of the clitoris is shaped like an upside-down "Y", or wishbone shape. Two legs – called crura – extend about 9cm (3½in) out from the clitoral body, encircling a pair of vestibular – or clitoral – bulbs, the whole structure wrapping around either side of the vaginal canal and the urethra. When we're aroused, the spongy erectile tissue that the structure is made up of becomes engorged with blood and swells in size – with some research showing that the entire clitoral complex reaches double its normal size. This

In a 2022 hospital waiting room survey, 37% of people mislabelled the clitoris.

reveals why the clitoris can be more easily stimulated internally when we're already turned on – explaining indirect stimulation via the vagina walls and "G-spot stimulation".

The clitoral erectile tissue is similar to that of the penis and has much the same function. This is because both the clitoris and penis develop from the same undifferentiated structure in the womb – the genital tubercle. When XX chromosomes are present, the tubercle usually transforms into the clitoris – though for some intersex people, the presence of XX sex chromosomes doesn't lead to the formation of a clitoris, and external genitalia appear more like a penis and testicles.

1 Clitoral glans
2 Crura
3 Vestibular bulbs
4 Urethral opening
5 Vagina

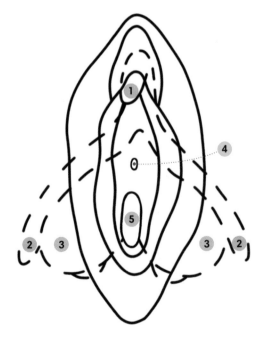

What about
the penis?

The penis and accompanying sex organs lie inside and outside of the body. External genitals comprise penis, testes, and scrotum; internal sex organs, the prostate, urethra, and vas deferens.

The external genitals

• **The penis** has the dual role of facilitating sex and urination, with both processes involving the urethra (see opposite). The penis – like the clitoris (see p.76) – originates from the structure called the genital tubercle in the fetus, which develops into a penis. Its structure is made up of the glans – the head, or end – and the shaft – the free part of the penis that connects to the body at the root and runs to the glans. Most of the nerve endings in the penis – it's thought around 4,000 – are densely packed into the penis glans, making this area highly sensitive. The glans is covered with the foreskin, a loose layer of skin that's removed in those who are circumcized. The shaft encloses three cylinders of spongy erectile tissue. One, the corpus spongiosum, houses the urethra; the other paired cylinders – the corpora cavernosa – play a key role in erections (see p.94).

    In its resting state the penis is referred to as flaccid. During arousal, it becomes temporarily engorged, causing it to stand upright and away from the body in an erect state. The skin covering the penis is loose enough to accommodate the changes that take place.

    For trans men who undergo bottom surgery (see p.83), external genitals are adopted to align with those of people assigned male at birth (AMAB). However, the penis created during a phalloplasty or metoidioplasty procedure doesn't produce sperm.

- **The frenulum** – the underside of the glans, between the shaft and foreskin – has the highest density of nerve endings. For some, this is the most sensitive part of the penis and is highly responsive to light touch.
- **The scrotum** is a sensitive fleshy sack that contains the testes, also known as testicles or balls. The oval-shaped testicles make sperm and produce testosterone. As the optimal temperature for sperm is slightly lower than body temperature, the scrotum sits outside the body for temperature control.

The internal genitals

- **The urethra** connects the bladder to the penis. It's involved in urination and carries semen – transported from the testes via the vas deferens – during ejaculation. Fluids leave at the urethral meatus – the penis tip.
- **The prostate** is a small gland between the bladder and penis. It produces seminal fluid that combines with sperm cells to make up semen. As it's surrounded by nerve endings, it can be stimulated for sexual pleasure (see p.85), either externally by massaging the perineum – the area between the anus and scrotum – or internally by anal penetration.

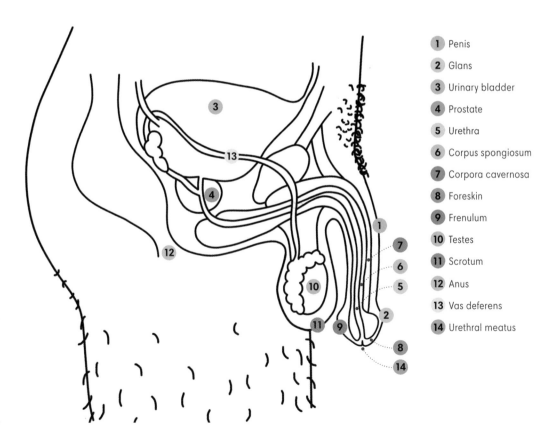

1. Penis
2. Glans
3. Urinary bladder
4. Prostate
5. Urethra
6. Corpus spongiosum
7. Corpora cavernosa
8. Foreskin
9. Frenulum
10. Testes
11. Scrotum
12. Anus
13. Vas deferens
14. Urethral meatus

Does size matter?

Penis anxiety can stem from skewed representations of genitalia and is also wrapped up in unhelpful cultural messaging connecting perceived masculinity to the size of a penis.

Commonplace jokes about shoe size relating to penis size – in fact an unreliable predictor of the size of a penis – can add to people with penises' feelings of insecurity about the size of their genitalia. One 2018 study that surveyed 200 heterosexual men found that penis size was a concern for 68 per cent of them. Another study by the UK charity LGBT HERO on 566 gay and bisexual men, found that 38 per cent had anxiety about their penis – with worries about it being either too small or too big – and that these anxieties sometimes had a knock-on impact on self-esteem.

Concerns about penis size, sometimes treated as trivial, can in fact influence the sexual satisfaction of those impacted, in some cases leading to performance anxiety and problems with sexual functioning. In turn, they can experience low sexual self-confidence – a predictor of less sexual satisfaction overall.

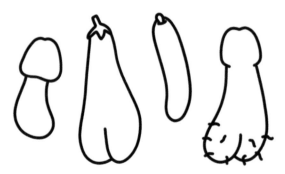

WHAT'S IN A MEASURE?

There's no consistent data on penis sizes. Some studies estimate the average flaccid penis is 9cm (3½in) in length and an erect one 12cm (5in). Data is largely drawn from self-measurement so is likely to be unreliable; in addition, flaccid penises are much more variable in size than erect ones, so studying them objectively is challenging.

Where does satisfaction lie?

While the comfort of people with their own bodies can fall prey to false messages about penis size and masculinity for those identifying as men, in reality there are so many facets of what it means to be a man that are unrelated to the size of one body part, with penis size far from the best measure of sexual satisfaction.

Pleasure given and received during sex is about far more than the size of genitalia. In terms of heterosexual penetrative sex, the fact that an orgasm gap exists between men and women (see p.170) is evidence that an erection and the requirement for this to be used for intercourse during sex in no way guarantees that your partner will orgasm. For the majority of people with a clitoris, the most direct route to orgasm is from clitoral stimulation, so forms of non-penetrative sex that don't require a penis or an erection are better predictors of pleasure and orgasm.

When asking women whether penis size mattered, one study found that 77 per cent described penis size as unimportant. Also, many gay and bisexual men report a preference for sexual acts other than anal penetration.

The size or shape of a penis has no bearing on the quality of a sexual partner, or the stamina that they may have for a sexual experience. Penis size also has no impact on the fertility of those assigned male at birth (AMAB), with sperm made in the testicles and its quality dependent on a variety of factors such as age and lifestyle.

Focusing on the pleasure you and your partner are experiencing, communicating what you like sexually, and accepting that all bodies are different, will make you more likely to enjoy sex and want to repeat the experience. Making adaptations to take into account what feels comfortable and works for us is part of sex. If worries about penis size feel difficult to put aside, consider the following:

• Stay curious and open. Try experimenting with positions to see what feels most comfortable for you and your partner.
• If you're concerned about the comfort of a larger penis for a partner, use lubricant and take things slowly.
• Embrace sex toys to make pleasure the main determinant of your satisfaction and take your focus away from worries about your body.

What can it mean to transition?

The umbrella term "trans" describes someone whose gender identity doesn't align with the sex they were assigned at birth.

Transitioning is the gender-affirming process that some trans people undergo to achieve their alignment of gender identity and sex assigned at birth and can be a hormonal, physical, social, psychological, and emotional experience. Multiple factors are at play, and there can be numerous barriers trans people face, which makes the process unique to each person and their circumstances.

Gender plays a big role in our lives, even if we identify as agender (see p.19), as it involves acceptance and being the person we know ourselves to be. It's well documented that transgender people, including non-binary people, can experience poorer mental health, likely due to stigma, discrimination, and a lack of social support and inclusion. Gender-affirming care is associated with an increase in wellbeing and better mental health.

Gender-affirming care encompasses transitioning, which can involve social, hormonal, and surgical processes, alongside supportive counselling. Each person can choose which changes to undergo and their timeline. Some find social changes enough

and that these can let them go at their own pace and for their gender expression to fluctuate if needed; others transition hormonally. Many surgical options require prior hormone therapy and for social transition to be established. Many feel that both top and bottom surgery (see opposite) isn't needed. For instance, many trans men find top surgery to remove breasts greatly reduces body dysphoria.

Social transition

Adopting new pronouns, changing a name, and exploring different clothing helps some to transition. Some trans men along with some non-binary people also practice chest binding to compress the breasts, ideally under the guidance of a trusted healthcare provider.

Hormonal transition

Done under medical supervision, this results in bodily changes – some, such as breast growth, are irreversible. For trans women, oestrogen therapy blocks testosterone, responsible for related secondary sex characteristics, such as tone of voice and body hair growth. It also affects sperm production and in turn fertility. Those transitioning report fewer erections, redistributed body fat, and breast growth. Oestrogen hormone therapy may also produce emotional and physical symptoms similar to premenstrual syndrome (PMS), or the more severe premenstrual dysphoric disorder (PMDD), without a menstrual bleed.

Testosterone therapy for trans men results in a deeper voice, increased facial hair, changes in muscle mass, and clitoral enlargement. The menstrual cycle is also suppressed so periods cease and some experience menopausal symptoms (see pp.234–235).

Surgical transition

Also called gender-affirmation/confirmation surgery, or gender-reassignment surgery, this can be the final stage of a physical transition after hormone therapy. It can involve multiple procedures and either/both bottom and top surgery to change the physicality and function of the chest and genitals. For trans women, external genitals can be reconstructed to form a neovulva and neovagina. The aim is for sensitivity to enable that person to enjoy the sex life they desire as the gender they know themselves to be. A neovagina produces little moisture, so lubricant is needed for sex.

For trans men, a phalloplasty or metoidioplasty can be done and a scrotum created. Phalloplasty involves several procedures to construct a neopenis of average size and urethra from tissue elsewhere, usually the arm or thigh. For a metoidioplasty, existing genital tissue is used to create a smaller neopenis, not always large enough for penetration, but able to become erect when aroused. With both procedures, ejaculation isn't possible, but orgasm is, though levels of sensation will vary for each person. Some trans men may choose to access a hysterectomy or oophorectomy.

Is the G spot real?

Anecdotally, around 63 per cent of women say they have a G spot, with many saying it brings pleasure. However, the existence of the G spot as a structure has been historically debated.

The G spot is named after the German scientist Ernst Gräfenburg, who in the 1950s claimed to have discovered an erotic spot on the anterior vaginal wall. With little subsequent research, the debate surrounding its existence has continued ever since.

Today, our understanding is that rather than being a precise anatomical structure, the G spot is a highly pleasurable zone in the front wall of the vagina and forms part of the clitoral network (see p.76). Clitoral tissue is more textured and spongy than the vaginal walls, becoming engorged when we're turned on; this means the G spot, or zone, is more pleasurable to stimulate when already aroused. It's best reached by inserting fingers into the vagina in a "come hither" motion to reach the anterior wall, which is why sex toys for G-spot stimulation are slightly curved. Certain partnered positions may also reach this area more easily (see pp.103–104).

Those assigned female at birth (AFAB) who experience pleasure this way describe it as an intense, deeper sensation than direct clitoral stimulation. However, it's helpful to bear in mind that the majority of people with a vulva don't orgasm from vaginal sex alone. When it comes to pleasure, the key thing is to explore what works for you – whether that's direct clitoral stimulation, vaginal stimulation, or simultaneous vaginal and clitoral stimulation – rather than feel pressure to discover a particular source of pleasure.

75% of women don't orgasm frequently from vaginal sex.

How do you stimulate the prostate?

Sometimes referred to as the male "G spot", or "P spot", this small gland located between the bladder and the penis is surrounded by sensitive nerve endings.

The prostate is one of several glands that produces fluid that combines with sperm to make up semen – or seminal fluid – released during ejaculation. As well as its reproductive role, the nerve endings around the prostate mean that it can be stimulated for pleasure. Those assigned male at birth (AMAB) and some intersex people, depending on their sexual characteristics, will have a prostate.

Accessing a source of pleasure

Any person with a prostate can experience a prostate orgasm, and prostate and anal play can give sexual pleasure regardless of gender identity or sexual orientation. Stimulating the prostate is a different way of incorporating pleasure into your sex life. For direct stimulation, the prostate is reached via anal penetration with the fingers or anal or prostate sex toys with a flared base (see p.58). A good-quality water-based lube is essential (see p.86) and nails should be trimmed to avoid damage to the anal cavity and prostate. As with any anal play, comfort, communication, and slowing the pace is key. If penetration via the anus isn't your preference, the prostate can be stimulated indirectly and externally by gently massaging the perineum with hands or a sex toy. Some toys stimulate the anus internally and the perineum at the same time.

The prostate is best stimulated when already aroused, when fluid for ejaculation causes it to swell. While clinical research on how prostate orgasms occur is lacking, anecdotally many report experiencing intense pleasure and a deeper orgasm, especially when combined with the sensations of anal penetration.

When should we use lube?

Lubrication can be used in almost any sexual situation and is an easy and accessible way to enhance our sex lives – whatever our genitals, sex, gender, or sexual orientation.

Lubricant reduces friction between touching body parts during sex, creating a slide or glide technique to make movements smoother, more comfortable, and ultimately more pleasurable. It's essential for anal sex (see opposite) and can be used generally during solo or partnered play. Lube should also be used with all sex toys and can increase sensitivity when used together.

There are also times when we may need to adapt our sex lives to include lubricant. For example, breastfeeding, menopause, and some medications can lead to vaginal dryness. Lube is helpful, too, for those assigned male at birth (AMAB) who've gone through gender-affirmation surgery. Choose a type to suit your needs – and avoid any lubes with harsh chemicals such as parabens and glycerine.

- **Water-based lubes** are condom- and sex toy-compatible. They wash off easily but can dry out quickly so repeat applications may be needed.

- **Oil-based lubes** feel more textured and are longer-lasting. However, they aren't condom- or sex toy-compatible as the oil can break down materials.
- **Silicone-based lube** has a soft, silky texture. It's also water-resistant so ideal for use in water, and is both condom- and sex-toy compatible.

DO YOU NEED TO WASH OFF LUBE?

This isn't vital so is down to personal preference. Some suggest it can avoid spreading bacteria that lead to UTIs; others feel leaving it on helps moisturize the genitals. When you do wash, avoid "hygiene" products marketed for genitals, which reinforce ideas about them being dirty.

- The slightly acidic vagina – pH 3.8–4.5 – is self-cleaning and has lactobacillus bacteria to protect against infection. Avoid soap or body wash as they can affect this environment.
- Wash the vulva and penis in warm water, using a little mild soap if you wish. Gently pull back the foreskin of the penis to wash under there.

How do we enjoy safe anal play?

Anal play is another way to give and receive pleasure in both partnered and solo sex. It can be part of anyone's sex life, regardless of gender and sexual orientation.

Densely packed with nerve endings and blood vessels, the anus is highly sensitive. It has thinner walls than the vagina so its tissues are more delicate. Ringed muscles form an internal and external sphincter. These contract strongly, playing a key part in bowel movements.

Anal play can involve penetration with the penis, a finger, or sex toys, and oral stimulation, known as rimming. In people assigned male at birth (AMAB), anal penetration is how the prostate is reached and stimulated (see p.85); for men who have sex with men, anal sex may play a key role, with partners choosing to be top or bottom, or switching. Some trans men and non-binary people might use a prosthetic or strap-on penis to penetrate a partner, and cis women can also explore this.

The anus doesn't self-lubricate sufficiently to support penetration so it's essential to use lube. Anal lubes are less acidic than vaginal ones. They also tend to be thicker, protecting delicate anal tissue to help prevent tearing that increases the risk of spreading STIs (see p.204). If using sex toys, it's important to choose ones

designed for anal play, such as butt plugs (see p.58), with a flared base. This ensures that during strong anal contractions, for example, when we orgasm, they aren't sucked up into the body's cavity. Ideally, start with a smaller toy to warm up and relax before using a bigger one.

Numbing agents should be avoided as discomfort is your guide on when to slow down. As you can't see where you're stimulating, communication with a partner is key to help you relax physically and psychologically. If exploring anal play for the first time, take your time and slow the pace or stop if it becomes painful.

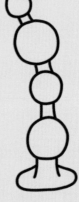

How does the brain sense touch?

Our brain interprets information about the world around us from nerve signals sent via the numerous nerve endings in the body's largest organ – our skin.

Our sense of touch is governed by the somatosensory system – a network of neurons that generate sensory-motor feedback between the body and brain. The brain's somatosensory cortex receives information about touch, pain, temperature, and pressure, localizing sensations; it also processes information on movement – called proprioception – making us aware of our body in relation to its surroundings.

Sensitive areas

The nerve endings in our skin that feed back to the somatosensory cortex aren't uniformly distributed around the body. In places where there's a greater density of nerve endings, such as the lips and fingertips, increased signals mean we feel sensations more intensely.

The organization of nerve endings and the corresponding area of the somatosensory cortex are also correlated. From the 1930s, neurosurgeon Dr Wilder Penfield carried out research on male epilepsy patients. He devised a map of the sensory cortex (see opposite), revealing how areas that have the highest density of nerve endings are allocated a larger part of the cortex, to process touch in that area.

Connecting touch

Our experience of touch is supported by our chemistry. The neurochemical oxytocin, which has a bonding effect (see p.111), is released in response to touch and physical intimacy, rewarding us for making human connections. Oxytocin also counteracts the effects of the stress hormone cortisol, promoting calmness, which in turn has a positive impact on health.

Research shows how our understanding of touch is critical to our connections with others. A study by psychologist Matthew Hertenstein separated participants by a barrier; with no other social information, such as hearing or sight, they were able to detect different emotions being communicated with only brief touches to the forearm 55–60 per cent of the time.

Individual perceptions

How we receive touch is also down to our personal makeup. Some describe "sensory overload", where an overstimulation of one or more of their senses feels overwhelming. This can happen to anyone and isn't uncommon in new parents or those breastfeeding, who can temporarily crave the sensation of space and the desire that demands aren't placed on their body. "Touch overload" is also more common in neurodivergent people, who may experience hypersensitivity, meaning that sensory input such as touch can feel intolerable. Their instinct may be to avoid rather than approach sex and intimacy; developing strategies to help enjoy touch more easily and communicating with partners can be helpful. Conversely, some neurodivergent people are less attuned to certain senses, known as hyposensitivity, and may need increased, or more intense, sensation to feel aroused.

MAPPING TOUCH SIGNALS

This map of the somatosensory cortex is based on the original by Dr Penfield. The longer the blue dash, the more space the brain gives to process touch from this area. The lips, for instance, although a small part of the body, are densely packed with nerve endings, so the brain allocates more space to process touch signals.

1. Somatosensory cortex

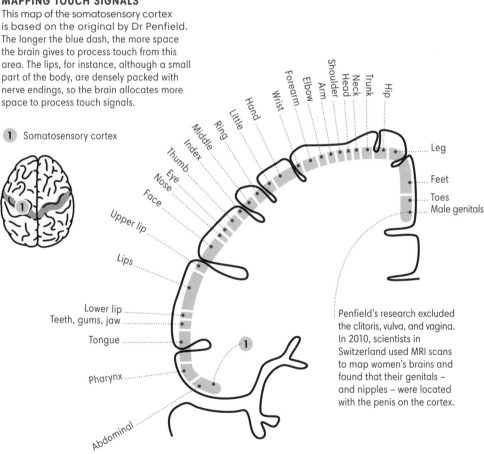

Penfield's research excluded the clitoris, vulva, and vagina. In 2010, scientists in Switzerland used MRI scans to map women's brains and found that their genitals – and nipples – were located with the penis on the cortex.

Do we all have the same erogenous zones?

The exploration of our erogenous zones through touch is not just a question of nerve endings – how we perceive and translate that touch is also influential.

Our erogenous zones are the parts of our bodies that elicit sexual feelings when touched. Studies have identified numerous extragenital erogenous zones – non-genital areas that arouse us when stimulated. A 2016 study found that the inner thigh, buttocks, lips, nipples, neck, ears, and breasts were key zones. In the same study, 12 per cent of women reported orgasm via stimulation of an extragenital zone. While areas with the highest density of sensory nerve structures, such as the lips and genitals, are often the most sensitive, in reality, any part of our skin – our largest sense organ – is a potential erogenous zone, depending on what feels pleasurable for each person.

Because our brains are adaptable – known as neuroplasticity – discovering a new erogenous zone can form new neural pathways, with repeated touch strengthening these pathways. The brain can also move functions from damaged areas to non-damaged areas, called functional plasticity. This means, for example, that some who've experienced a spinal cord injury are potentially able to hone sensitivity to other areas of the body, creating new pleasure-giving zones.

Our brains can also transmit messages about how touch feels socially and emotionally, which can affect how we experience touch. For example, if someone touches us too soon, or we perceive touch as threatening, our brain signals our preference not to be touched, even if this is in a pleasurable area.

BODY-MAPPING EXERCISE

Take some time, without distraction, to focus on the sensation of touch. Slowly explore your body from head to toe, noticing which areas feel more or less sensitive. When you find a spot you like, try different touch styles, for example, with the flat of your hand or fingertips; with softer or firmer pressure, or a slower or faster stroke. Exploring in this way can expand your sexual repertoire, introducing different types of touch to areas of the body you might not usually focus on during sex.

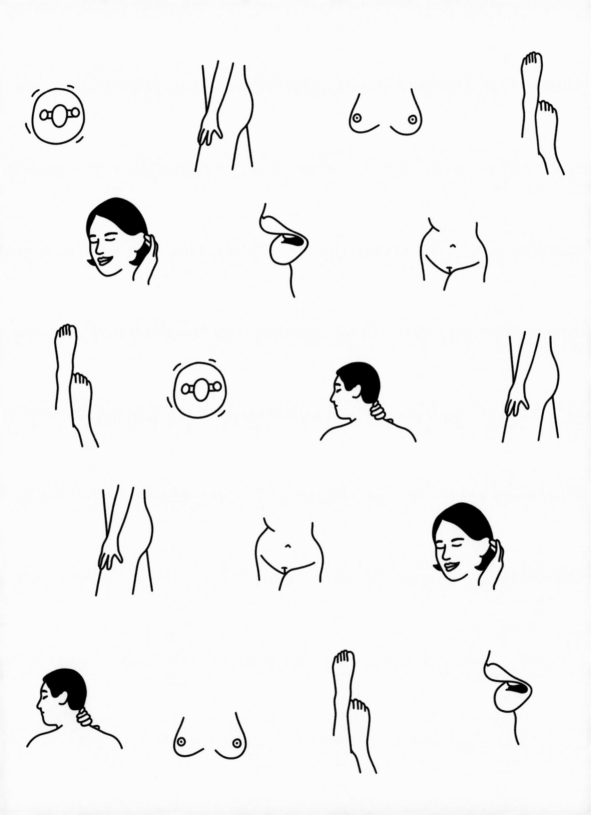

What happens when
we're **aroused?**

Our understanding of exactly what happens in our bodies and minds during sex has evolved in recent decades as we've come to appreciate the role that desire plays in sexual response.

Arousal is the feeling of being turned on sexually. Many experience this as a change in how our bodies, and particularly our genitals, feel. It's caused by the brain sending messages to prepare the body for sexual activity. An increased blood flow to the genitals can create a boost in sensitivity and swelling, which can be felt as the start of an erection for people with penises, or, for those with a vagina, an increase in wetness.

In the 1960s, pioneering sexologists Masters and Johnson presented a four-phase model for sexual arousal: excitement, plateau, orgasm, and resolution. This linear model set out the physiological processes our bodies go through during sex:

- **In the excitement phase**, sexual stimuli causes the physical and physiological responses described opposite, such as increased breathing, blood flow, and heart rate and a build up of muscle tension.
- **In the plateau phase** – the lead up to orgasm – excitement and sensitivity intensifies.

- **Orgasm** is the peak of sexual pleasure (see p.96).
- **In the resolution phase**, the muscles relax, breathing and heart rate decrease, and the genitals return to their pre-excited state.

How thinking has evolved

Masters and Johnson's model accurately set out what happens to our bodies during sex. However, it's now understood that this linear model is limited as it takes into account the physical aspects of sex only and, especially for women, discounts that orgasm isn't always a part of sex. We now understand that sex can't be separated from desire (see p.130) and that we can feel psychologically or cognitively turned on. So sex and desire are context-dependent, with our environment playing a part in how we experience arousal (see p.158).

What's consistent across modern sexuality research is that the more concordance – or synchronicity – we have between body and mind, the stronger our sexual response is likely to be.

Increased blood flow to the genitals during arousal prepares the body for sex.

The sexual response process

When aroused, physiological processes occur, some of which cause physical changes. During the arousal process of women and those assigned female at birth (AFAB):

- **Sexual stimuli triggers the brain** to send nerve messages to increase blood flow to the genitals. This can cause the labia and vagina to darken and they swell, which causes fluid to pass through the vaginal walls and increase lubrication (see p.74), building sensitivity for all types of sex. The clitoris engorges, becoming more sensitive, and retracts under its hood.
- **Breathing quickens** and the heart rate and blood pressure increase.
- **Neurochemicals are released** that cause blood vessels to dilate, and body temperature may rise. These can create a sex "flush" – a reddening of the skin – which can also be caused by skin-on-skin friction.
- **The nipples** may become erect.
- **The uterus lifts up** in the process called tenting (see p.74), creating more space in the vagina in preparation for penetration.
- **Muscle tension increases** in different parts of the body, but particularly in the pelvic floor muscles (see p.112) and the vagina-supporting pubococcygeus muscle.

During the arousal process of men and those assigned male at birth (AMAB):

- **The brain responds to sexual stimuli** and nerve messages cause the muscles of the corpora cavernosa – the two cylinders of spongy erectile tissue in the penis shaft – to relax, allowing blood to flow in and fill the tissues, leading to an erection (see p.94). Erections can fluctuate during sexual activity and the penis doesn't need to be fully hard and erect for the entire duration of a sexual experience for it to be satisfying and pleasurable. Some men lose erections completely then regain them.
- **Breathing quickens** and the heart rate and blood pressure increase.
- **Neurochemicals are released** that cause blood vessels to dilate, and body temperature may rise, which can create a sex "flush".
- **The nipples** may become erect.
- **Some men experience pre-ejaculate**, commonly known as "pre-cum" – an involuntary release of liquid from the penis before the point of ejaculation.

How do erections happen?

An erection is much more than a biological event – it requires the brain, body, and mind to all be on side.

Erections occur when the spongy tissue in the cylinders of the penis shaft – the corpora cavernosa - fill with blood, compressing the network of penile veins and causing the penis to harden and stand erect. This simple vascular event is the result of a complex chain reaction that starts in the brain, communicating to the penis via hormones and the spinal cord and nerves. During arousal, the hypothalamus releases testosterone, which helps coordinate erections with sex. Part of the hypothalamus – the paraventricular nucleus – fires messages between the brain and spinal cord, triggering the release of oxytocin and dopamine, a key neurotransmitter for facilitating erections. Nerve messages also activate the release of nitric oxide. This relaxes smooth tissue in the corpora cavernosa, allowing the penis to fill with blood.

There are two types of erection – psychogenic and reflexogenic. Psychogenic ones occur when the brain responds to sexually relevant stimuli. Reflexogenic result from direct penile stimulation. Not all people with penises can achieve both types. For example, for some with spinal cord injuries, a psychogenic erection may not be possible, but, dependent on the injury, a reflexogenic one may be (see p.122).

The whole process is controlled by the autonomic nervous system so, like breathing and digestion, arousal happens without our conscious control. This means that during arousal, excitatory signals can be interrupted by factors such as stress or distraction, sending the brain into fight-or-flight mode. This directs blood away from the penis to other parts of the body, leading to challenges such as erectile dysfunction (see p.122).

Up in the night

Erections also happen during sleep - known as nocturnal penile tumescene, or nocturnal erections – when you're not consciously interacting with stimuli. Occurring mostly in REM sleep, they're thought to help oxygenate penile tissue. It's normal to wake up with an erection, too, a phenomenon that decreases with age. While disrupted sleep or stress can interrupt morning erections, it's worth seeking medical advice if they suddenly no longer occur as this can indicate a potential health issue.

The myths around erections

There are many myths and flawed messages around erections. These include beliefs that men should always be ready and able to "get it up", that the ability to get an erection is linked to masculinity, and worries that problems with an erection mean you can't satisfy a partner. These reductive views of masculinity fail to take into account that each sexual situation is context-dependent, with factors such as emotional states playing a role. They also fail to recognize that there are many other ways to enjoy sexual pleasure beyond penetration and that intercourse isn't always the best route to sexually satisfying experiences for everyone.

CAN EVERYONE GET ERECTIONS?

Yes, like the penis, the clitoris is made up of erectile tissue (see p.76). In the clitoris, two areas of spongy erectile tissue, the corpora cavernosa, connect to the clitoral glans (tip). These fill with blood and enlarge during sex, increasing in sensitivity.

THE FLACCID PENIS

When unaroused, an equal amount of blood flows in and out of the penis and the penis remains soft and flaccid.

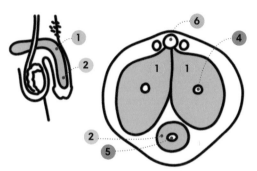

Cross-section of flaccid penis

1. Corpora cavernosa
2. Corpus spongiosum
3. Increased blood flow
4. Artery
5. Urethra
6. Veins

THE ERECTION PROCESS

When aroused, blood rushes to the penis, causing the corpus cavernosa vessels to compress, as shown in this cross section. Blood is trapped and the penis grows, hardens, and becomes erect.

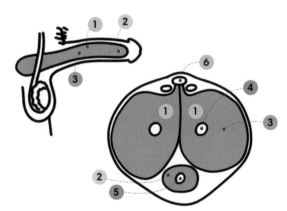

Cross-section of erect penis

What happens when we orgasm?

An orgasm is a peak body and brain pleasure experience. Involving our emotions and chain reactions in several body systems, they're often described as "mind-blowing" for a reason.

At the point of orgasm, the muscle tension that built up during the arousal process (see p.93) is followed by a discharge of involuntary rhythmic muscular spasms in the pelvis, causing contractions in the walls of the vagina, uterus, and anus in people with a vulva, and in the urethra and anus in people with a penis. This creates the sense of a pleasurable wave through the genitals and pelvis, and sometimes elsewhere. The heart, breathing rate, and blood pressure continue to rise steadily during the arousal process through to orgasm.

The role of the brain

The process of sexual arousal that can lead to orgasm is made up of a complex series of reactions in our hormones and circulatory and nervous systems. As sex is a multi-sensory process, numerous areas of the brain are activated during arousal. Studies with MRI scans by behavioural neuroscientist Barry R. Komisaruk revealed a surge of activity overwhelming the brain at the point of orgasm.

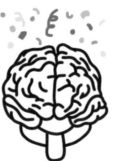

Almost as soon as we start a sexual act, the genital-sensory cortex becomes more active. The MRI scans studied by Komisaruk and his team also revealed that the vagina, cervix, and clitoris were associated with stimulation in different parts of the cortex, which the researchers suggested could add to the intensity of an orgasm if more than one area was stimulated at once. The genital-sensory cortex was also activated during nipple stimulation in women, which could help explain why some women orgasm this way.

- **The lateral orbitofrontal cortex** – the part of the brain associated with decision-making and reason – becomes less active during sex. This reduces feelings of anxiety and fear, both of which can interrupt arousal. Many people report a feeling of losing inhibitions and fully letting go during an intense sexual experience so this may be partly thanks to the suppression of this area.
- **The hippocampus** – the part of the brain involved in learning and memory – is activated during arousal and orgasm. This can impact how we assign meaning to sexual experiences or build up associations between sensory input such as smells or sights. So where a sight or smell, for example, is associated with a previous pleasurable sexual experience,

being exposed to this stimuli again during sex may help intensify arousal and orgasm as our brains make connections with previous erotic experiences.

- **The hypothalamus** is the part of our brain that links our endocrine and nervous systems, both critical to sex. At orgasm, this is responsible for a surge of oxytocin and dopamine, the feel-good neurochemicals that promote feelings of closeness and relaxation. Prolactin is also released, which can give us the satisfied, sleepy feeling often felt after orgasm.

During orgasm, our brains and bodies constantly fire messages between them as excitement builds.

Are there different types of orgasm?

While we can enjoy orgasm from a variety of experiences, the pleasure we feel is based on a number of factors, such as speed, pressure, and, most importantly, context.

The stimulation of different parts of the body – most commonly the genitals, and, for some, erogenous zones such as the nipples – can bring us to orgasm. When thinking about "types" of orgasm, it's important to bear in mind that, while the right amount of stimulation in the right place can help us orgasm, our psychology and the subjectivity of our experience play a critical part.

- **Blended orgasms** can occur when different areas are stimulated at once, such as the nipples and clitoris.
- **Multiple orgasms** are a succession of orgasms in a short period of time. They're most common in people with a vulva as there's no refractory period (see p.101), but anyone can experience them. Some find the genitals too sensitive after orgasm to touch. For others, continued stimulation can create a wave of orgasms, which, as the body is already in an aroused state, may happen more easily than the initial one.
- **Simultaneous orgasms** are when we orgasm at the same time as a partner. Though not more intense, they can feel connecting; however, they are not a criteria for good sex.
- **Nocturnal orgasms** occur during sleep, when we're relaxed and blood flow around the body is increased.
- **"Breath" orgasms** are a type of hands-free orgasm. This uses breathing to focus attention on pleasurable sensations and takes practice.

THE ORGASM SOCK DEBATE

A 2015 study found that, when wearing socks, 80 per cent of participants orgasmed, compared to 50 per cent when not wearing socks. Theories for why included cold feet being a distraction and socks increasing circulation, which helps arousal. But for many, wearing socks was a turn off, so it's really an individual preference!

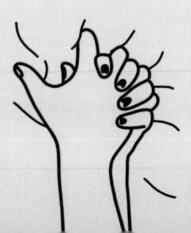

Why is it taking me so long to orgasm?

Preoccupation with time is linked to what we feel is expected of us sexually and can become a distraction. Redirecting our focus away from orgasm and onto our sensations can prove helpful.

Worries about taking too long to orgasm are often linked to our situation. For example, some find it easier to climax during solo rather than partnered sex. This may be because we aren't receiving, or communicating, the physical stimulation we need to orgasm, or because we're struggling to relax psychologically.

Society places so much emphasis on orgasm. This can make us feel as though we have a problem if we don't orgasm and can leave us and our partners with a sense that sex, even if perfectly enjoyable, was unsatisfactory because we didn't climax. In fact, the more orgasm becomes a goal, the less likely we are to reach it. Focusing on the goal takes us away from experiencing the pleasurable sensations that are most likely to get us to peak pleasure. We can also fall into a negative cycle where worries about orgasm not happening create performance anxiety, keeping us in an anxious rather than aroused state and distracting us from the pleasure that takes us to orgasm.

If you're struggling to orgasm, clear communication about what feels good for you, and avoiding thinking of orgasm as a direct measure of sex or that there's a time limit on reaching it, can help you focus your attention on what feels good for you.

We've been socialized to think that sex without an orgasm is a failure.

What happens during ejaculation?

Ejaculation happens at the peak of sexual excitement. It's a reflex action – so once you reach this moment there's no going back.

Ejaculation – an involuntary reflex controlled by the autonomic nervous system – is the expulsion of fluid during sex. Ejaculation and orgasm are often thought of as one event but are actually two separate processes that commonly, but don't always, happen together – sometimes orgasm can happen without ejaculating, known as a dry orgasm.

There are two phases to ejaculation – emission and expulsion. At the peak of excitement, the emission stage prepares semen and closes the bladder neck to stop semen entering the bladder. In the expulsion phase, rhythmic contractions of the pelvic floor muscles propel semen along the urethra and eject it out of the body via the urethra meatus (see p.79). Rarely, semen does enter the bladder, known as retrograde ejaculation. This isn't harmful but may cause distress and can be a problem when trying to conceive, in which case fertility treatment may be needed.

THE PATH OF SPERM
At ejaculation, sperm is forced from the epididymis into the vas deferens. It combines with seminal fluid and travels via the prostate to the urethra, where it's ejaculated via the urethral meatus.

1. Epididymis
2. Vas deferens
3. Seminal vesicles
4. Prostate
5. Urethra
6. Urethral meatus

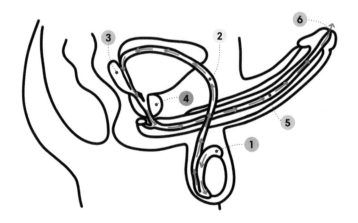

How **soon** can I orgasm again?

The idea of multiple orgasms may sound appealing, but a recovery stage after climax means that often this isn't an option.

Where is ejaculate made?

Ejaculate is made up of sperm cells and seminal fluid. The vast majority of ejaculate – around 70 per cent – comes from the seminal vesicles. The rest comprises sperm cells from the testicles, along with fluid from the prostate and the bulbourethral, or Cowper's, glands. This means that those who undergo a vasectomy, where the vas deferens is cut, sealed, or blocked, are unlikely to notice a change in the amount of ejaculate.

What about squirting?

There's much fascination and not enough research on the topic commonly known as "female ejaculation". Some people with vulvas report squirting, or releasing, fluid at the point of climax. It's thought that the fluid is a combination of urine and a milky white fluid released from the Skene's glands (see p.75). This happens regularly for some women, while others never experience it. However, being preoccupied with or too focused on the idea of squirting happening is likely to distract you from your overall pleasure.

The time between an orgasm and when we're able to be sexually aroused again is called the refractory period.

In those assigned male at birth (AMAB), typically the penis is physically unable to become erect for a period of time after ejaculation. There are many factors, including health and age, that impact the length of time this takes, and it varies from person to person and between sexual experiences. Typically, the refractory period for men increases with age – for younger men, it may be just a few minutes; for older men it can be up to 24 hours or longer.

Those assigned female at birth (AFAB) don't have refractory periods in the same way as people with penises, so in theory can have multiple orgasms. However, some may find the genitals feel too sensitive post-orgasm to want to continue (which can be the case for people with a penis, too), and/or may feel physical and psychological fatigue, which dampens their interest in sex for a time. Everyone has a resolution period, when the body returns to its pre-arousal state (see p.92).

Do **positions** make a difference?

Sex positions can be adapted to suit our moods, energy levels, abilities, and desires. Exploring favourite positions or trying something new can increase our motivation for sex.

Missionary position

The bottom partner lies on their back, with the top partner lying between their legs.

Good for: eye contact and intimacy. Sex toys can be incorporated.

Adaptations: placing a pillow beneath the hips of a partner with a clitoris can create more clitoral contact. For many couples, it can be adapted to focus on clitoral stimulation, called the coital alignment technique. The top partner is higher, their chest in line with their partner's shoulders, and the bodies closer, changing the motion from thrusting to rubbing and grinding, putting more pleasurable pressure on the clitoris. For couples where both partners have a penis, the bottom partner lifts the legs higher for anal penetration.

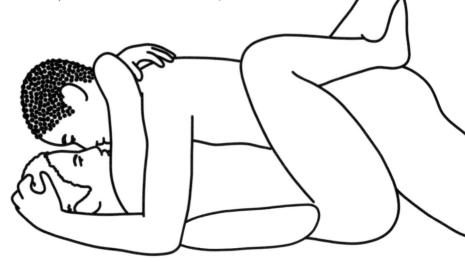

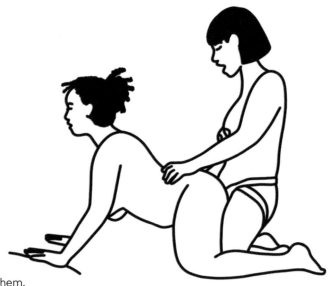

Doggy position

With one partner on all-fours, the other kneels behind to penetrate them.

Good for: deep penetration and G spot stimulation, and if you're not in the mood for sex with lots of eye contact.

Adaptations: a strap-on can be used, and the angle can be adjusted for anal penetration. The angle of the body of the partner in front can be changed by lowering the forearms so that the front of the body is lower and the hips are higher; or the receiving partner can position themselves over the side of a bed, which can change the sensations.

Exploration can add novelty and enhance pleasure.

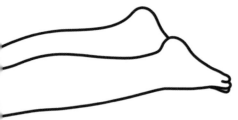

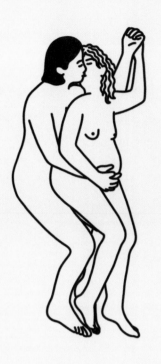

Spooning

Couples lie on their sides facing the same way, the partner behind pressing against the other's back. The front partner is nicknamed the "little spoon", the partner behind "big spoon".

Good for: slow and more gentle, less energetic sex, with or without penetration. It's great for mutual masturbation; all-over body exploration, including genital touch; kissing; and for using sex toys. Penetration at an angle can stimulate the G spot. Also good for pregnancy as it doesn't put pressure on the stomach.

Adaptations: both partners can change the position of their legs to alter the angle, which can offer deeper penetration and more intense thrusting.

Mutual masturbation

Partners touch and play with each other's genitals simultaneously; or self-pleasure in each other's presence.

Good for: those who aren't able to, or don't wish to, have intercourse. It's very visual so you can witness your partner's pleasure, and by moving away from penetration it can focus on clitoral touch.

Adaptations: this can be adjusted as desired based on ability, body type, comfort, energy levels, and location. Sex toys and lubricant add new sensations and ways of exploring.

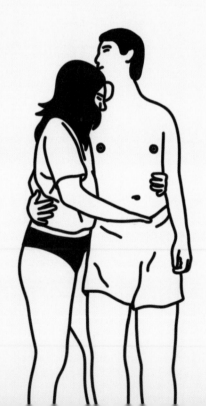

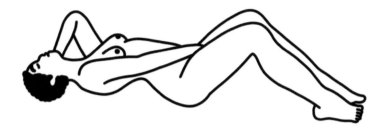

Solo sex

As the name suggests, this is about self-pleasure and sexual experiences without a partner. The human body is designed for pleasure and we all have different preferences and desires, so masturbation can be completely tailored by you for whatever you desire at that time.

Good for: self-exploration, getting to know your body, and self-focused pleasure.

Adaptations: you can use sex toys, lubricant, and stimulation such as erotica or porn. Try different locations, for example, self-pleasure in the shower, or change your body position.

Outercourse

Essentially, this is sexual activity without penetration. Importantly, the term is a departure from the word foreplay, recognizing that non-penetrative touch is not always a precursor to intercourse, but a pleasurable event in itself.

Good for: all bodies; for breaking out of routines – focusing on pleasure and what feels good, rather than something that you think you should be doing.

Adaptations: it can be adapted as wished and can involve dry-humping, grinding, touching, sex toys, massage, mutual masturbation (see opposite), and oral sex.

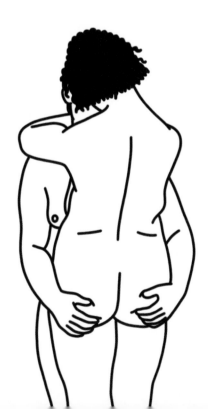

Can **menstrual hormones** affect libido?

Menstrual hormones can causes fluctuations in libido. However, our responses are individual and other factors can come into play.

Hormones – the body's chemical messengers – are released into the bloodstream by endocrine glands. They work in a delicately balanced feedback system to keep body systems steady and functioning, while also playing a part in our emotional equilibrium.

Our motivation for sex is very much context dependent, being influenced by any number of external factors (see p.158). However, the rise and fall of the two key sex hormones in the menstrual cycle – oestrogen and progesterone – can play a role in libido, together with a small amount of testosterone (see p.108).

The role of oestrogen in libido

From puberty to menopause, oestrogen plays a central role in reproductive and vaginal health. It's produced primarily by the ovaries, but fat cells and the adrenal glands also make small amounts. Oestrogen therapy is also part of a hormonal transition for trans women. During the menstrual cycle, around ovulation, levels of oestrogen – and testosterone – rise. As oestrogen rises, typically this is followed in the next day or so by increased vaginal lubrication, and, in turn, greater genital sensitivity. Noticing an increase in lubrication can in itself turn our thoughts to sex, triggering arousal and

Hormonal changes can influence how we feel and may lead to temporary changes in desire.

corresponding desire. While a rise in desire isn't scientifically proven, some scientists suggest that as ovulation is the time of peak fertility, these physical changes make evolutionary sense, maximizing the chance of conception.

Progesterone and desire

This hormone is key for maintaining the uterine lining in pregnancy, with levels rising after ovulation to prepare the womb for a fertilized egg. Anecdotally, women report a fall in libido when progesterone is highest – after ovulation, in the luteal phase of the menstrual cycle.

The luteal phase – between ovulation and a period – is when many report premenstrual syndrome (PMS) – a combination of emotional and physical symptoms, such as mood swings, poor concentration, anxiety, and breast tenderness, which can be hard to untangle. PMS can be most prominent just before a period, when both oestrogen and progesterone levels drop. The symptoms and their intensity vary widely; for some, their psychological and physical impact decreases their motivation for sex.

MENSTRUAL HORMONES AND LIBIDO
Being aware of how the rise and fall of hormones in our menstrual cycles can impact desire can help us understand potential reasons for why we might not feel "in the mood".

1 **Oestradiol**
Shortly after oestradiol – a key oestrogen – rises, lubrication and sensitivity increase, which can boost libido in the days before ovulation at about day 14.

2 **Progesterone**
When progesterone is high, libido typically drops. Symptoms such as bloating, along with PMS, can dampen desire.

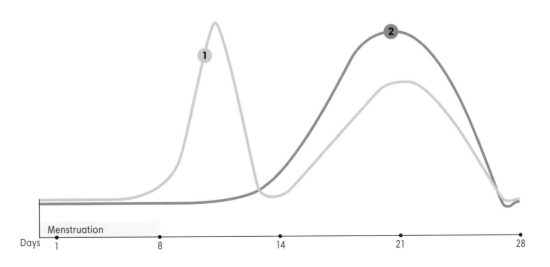

Menstruation

Days 1   8   14   21   28

Does testosterone impact sex?

Testosterone, a key sex hormone, plays a central role in sexual desire and functioning for men. It also impacts women's libido, but to a lesser extent.

Testosterone is produced mainly in the testes for men and those assigned male at birth (AMAB), where it plays an important role in sperm production; for women and those assigned female at birth (AFAB), the ovaries produce testosterone. The adrenal glands also produce testosterone for all sexes. Testosterone therapy can be part of the transitioning process for trans men if they choose this, prompting the onset of secondary sex characteristics (see p.83).

Testosterone and desire

This key sex hormone is thought to play an important role in sex drive. Although its impact isn't fully understood, reduced levels are associated with a lower motivation for sex. In a 2006 US study asking 1,500 men about their sex desire, those reporting low libido had correlating lower levels of testosterone.

For women and AFAB people, a balance of oestrogen and a little testosterone is important. It's thought that just small amounts of testosterone are needed to help maintain mood and sexual libido for these groups, who have on average around one-tenth to two-tenths the amount of testosterone as men.

Sexual function and testosterone

Aside from desire, testosterone is key for the sexual function of men and AMAB people. In the brain, it plays a central part in the synthesis of the neurotransmitters involved with erections, namely nitric oxide, oxytocin, and dopamine, which in turn help coordinate the physiological events that lead to an erection (see p.94).

Low testosterone levels can be associated with erection issues (see p.122). Other related factors can also contribute to sexual dysfunction. For example, there's a well-documented link between low testosterone and obesity, with both linked to erectile dysfunction. Moreover, some symptoms of low testosterone, such as fatigue, low mood, declined interest in sex, and erectile dysfunction, interlink with social factors such as relationship wellbeing, body confidence, self-esteem, and performance anxiety. It's important, therefore, to consider that multiple factors can be at play. Medical conditions associated with raised levels of testosterone, such as polycystic ovary syndrome (PCOS) in AFAB people, can impact both libido and fertility.

Can exercise boost testosterone?

Testosterone levels rise temporarily after exercise, especially after intense strength training, and increased muscle is linked with higher testosterone levels. However, excessive exercise without adequate rest is actually linked to lower testosterone levels in all genders.

A study showed that testosterone levels in new dads fell by an average of 34%.

TESTOSTERONE LEVELS
Normal testosterone levels in men are 10–35 nmol/l (300–1,000 ng/dl); in women, 0.5–2.4 nmol/l (15–70 ng/dl) is the average.

Men and those AMAB
Testosterone peaks around the age of 19; levels start to decline more rapidly at 30–40 years old, dropping about 2 per cent a year.

Women and those AFAB
Levels peak around the age of 19 then decline gradually, with a further drop around menopause.

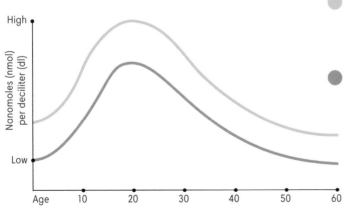

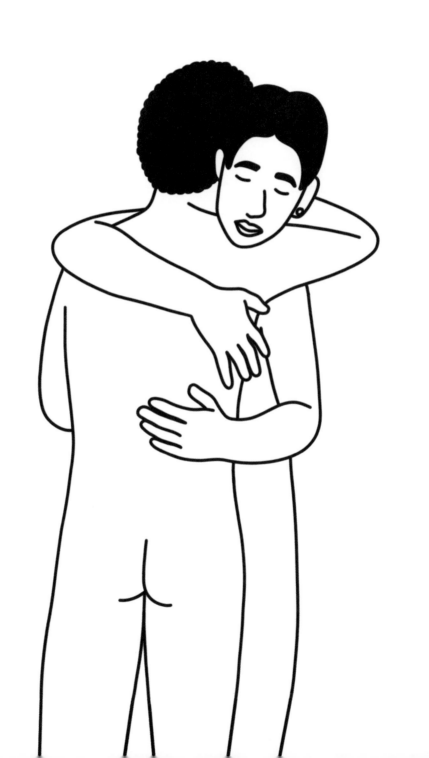

Are there "love" hormones?

As well as our sex hormones, our brains produce hormones that also act as neurotransmitters. Some of these chemicals can affect our emotions and how we feel during sex.

Often referred to as our "happy hormones", neurotransmitters dopamine and oxytocin, produced by the hypothalamus, have a significant impact on how we experience sex and pleasure. These two hormones can work synergistically, working together to enhance each others' effects. Dopamine production is stimulated and increased by the release of oxytocin, which is itself released when we are enjoying the sensation of touch. The release of dopamine – the reward-seeking hormone (see p.56) – motivates us to continue with pleasurable activities such as sex. We are then rewarded with a surge of additional neurochemicals during sex and orgasm, including oxytocin.

- Released during sexual or intimate interactions such as kissing, touch, and hugging, oxytocin is often nicknamed the cuddle hormone as it plays a role in social bonding, touch, and closeness. This is the hormone responsible for what people describe as a "warm, fuzzy feeling" during sex. When we orgasm we get an extra surge of oxytocin, which could be a biological reason for why couples often describe feeling closer after sex.
- Dopamine plays a big role in reward, and therefore in motivation. It's produced in response to sexual stimulation and is associated with pleasure and anticipating pleasure. As with oxytocin, our bodies receive a big surge of dopamine when we climax, motivating us to repeat this rewarding experience.

Can pelvic floor exercises improve sex?

The group of hammock-like muscles known as the pelvic floor stretch from the pubic bone to the coccyx. As well as supporting the bladder and bowel, they play a role in sex for everyone.

Pelvic floor exercises are most commonly discussed during pregnancy and the postnatal period. However, keeping this important group of muscles in shape can have unexpected benefits for our sex lives across all genders and ages.

How does the pelvic floor help sex?

The pelvic floor muscles assist with erections, ejaculation, and penetration. A toned pelvic floor also promotes healthy blood flow to the pelvic area and genitals, increasing sensitivity overall.

For people with a penis, a toned pelvic floor helps to manage blood flow to the penis, key to the erection process. Once erect, being able to recognize how and when to control the muscles involved in ejaculation offers a window of opportunity to control your pleasure up to just before the point of ejaculation, which is a reflex reaction.

For people with a vulva, the pelvic floor plays a role in comfortable penetration as the vaginal canal passes through the pelvic floor. In its resting state, the vagina is like a flattened tube. A toned pelvic floor supports the expansion of the vagina during penetration. However, if the pelvic floor is too tight, known as a hypertonic pelvic floor, this can create tension, leading to resistance to penetration and uncomfortable intercourse. Being able to relax the pelvic floor is therefore as important as being able to tense it – the key is to find a balance.

What about orgasms?

Part of orgasm is the rhythmical muscular contractions of the pelvic floor, along with the muscles in the vagina, anus, and uterus. This means that the stronger these muscles, the more intensely we can experience the pleasurable sensations.

One study correlated a toned pelvic floor with higher levels of sexual function.

IDENTIFYING YOUR PELVIC FLOOR

For people of all genders, the best way to locate your pelvic floor muscles is to imagine that you're trying to stop passing urine, and simultaneously stop yourself passing wind. You should feel a sense of squeezing up and inwards, but without holding your breath or tightening your stomach, buttocks, or thighs. Ideally, do this about 10 times around three times a day. You can practise quickly tensing and releasing the muscles; then, as you get used to the exercise, hold the muscles for a few seconds – taking care not to overdo it.

- Start by doing exercises lying on your back or on your side with a pillow between your legs if this helps you feel comfortable.
- Progress to practising while sitting or standing, where gravity will challenge your muscles more. If you struggle to feel your pelvic muscles when lying down, doing exercises while upright may be easier.

Will my partner like my body?

Our ability to celebrate our bodies and what they do – our body confidence – is often overshadowed by negative societal messaging.

One of our biggest barriers to confidence is self-doubt. When it comes to our sex lives this can have a big impact, leading us to feel self-conscious and critical about our bodies. A common worry, often exacerbated by cultural messaging, is whether a partner will like our body – how it looks, feels, smells, and tastes. Harsh self-judgment can be a protection against rejection, the theory being that if we criticize ourselves it hurts less if a partner does so – but internalizing negative thoughts has a detrimental effect on wellbeing.

Self-doubt activates the body's fight-or-flight "threat" system, triggering the brain to release cortisol. In the context of sex, this can lead to avoidance behaviours to manage our sex lives and stave off a threat. So we might turn the light off so we can't be seen; avoid certain practices or positions, such as oral sex, or being on top if we feel this is less flattering; or avoid sex altogether.

To turn this around, we need to recognize that how we talk to ourselves – our inner voice – matters. Thanks to neural plasticity – the ability of our brains to change and adapt – learning how to manage negative feelings can help us overcome self-doubt. When we build positive messages around our bodies (see p.116), we activate two other emotional systems. Our "drive" system, which anticipates the release of the reward chemical dopamine, springs into action, motivating us to challenge negative messaging. In addition, our "mammalian" caregiving system is activated; this releases oxytocin, helping us to feel compassionate towards ourselves. Practising self-kindness therefore strengthens the neural pathways that challenge our inclination to self-doubt.

A DISTORTED VIEW

For some, worries about their body escalate and they fixate on self-perceived flaws in a part of the body, such as their face, skin, or, for some, their genitals. Called body dysmorphia, this condition can significantly impact sex, with distracting thoughts about the body affecting the ability to be in the moment and fully enjoy a sexual experience.

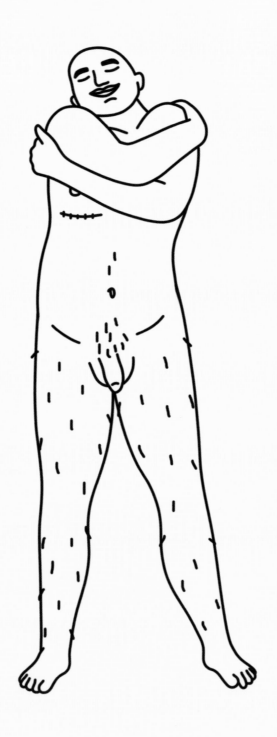

Can we learn to love our bodies?

Representations of the body in culture and social media often lack diversity, with body type trends dictating what's desirable at any one time. Too often this leads many to feel they don't "fit in".

Generally, familiarity with something helps us to build our confidence. However, when it comes to our bodies, especially our sexual bodies, it can feel that familiarity is discouraged. We pick up and start to internalize messages from a young age as we experience how others comment on and talk about bodies.

There are ways we can nurture our relationship with our bodies to build our body confidence. While some of these suggestions may feel alien at first, repeating an action helps our brains to habituate it.

Integrating some or all of the following practices into your day can form healthy habits that enhance wellbeing.

• **Practise daily affirmations** to challenge self-limiting and negative thoughts. Research shows that affirmation activates the brain's reward centres (see p.56). Your brain creates a mental image and repetition solidifies these cognitive thought patterns – in essence, you hear what you say and your brain responds. Offer daily affirmations

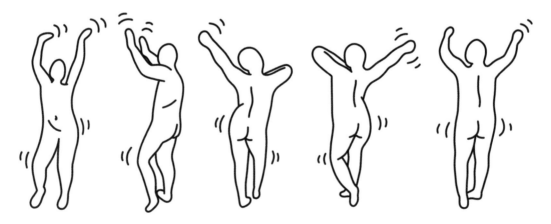

about your body, appreciating what your body can do. Grounding statements based in the present can help you accept that body positivity may fluctuate day to day.

- **Focus on movement** to experience your body in different ways. Movement also releases endorphins to trigger positive feelings. Notice muscles stretching or the sensation of air on your skin. Dance, exercise, and walking all help us to experience ourselves physically.
- **Practice mindful moisturizing**. Spend 10 minutes massaging a cream that you enjoy using into your skin. Focusing fully on the sensations can increase self-connection with your body, helping you associate your body with pleasure and lean into sensuality.
- **Resist placing value** or judgment on others' bodies, whether observing them in person or via visual images. Our instinct is to compare and see how we measure up, often with a self-negative bias. Observing others from a neutral position rather than an opinion-based one helps us to avoid this tendency.
- **Get comfortable with your body**. If there are areas you feel less comfortable with, such as your vulva, spend time simply holding your hand there, without masturbating.

I feel good in my body as it is today.

My body gives me pleasure.

I accept my body as it is.

The concept of body neutrality

Eating disorder specialist Anne Poirer, author of *The Body Joyful*, developed the concept of body neutrality. This arose as a response to the gaping distance between body negativity and positivity, offering a middle ground for those who struggle to make body positivity work. Some people feel pressure when asked to love their body, but need help to steer away from a negative body image. Body neutrality offers an approach grounded in respect and acceptance. The aim is to focus on what your body can do and how it makes you feel, rather than on how it looks, and to accept your body the way it is. This can help us to become less preoccupied with the value often placed on our bodies. This is helpful for some, especially those who feel that body confidence is a big leap that's not in-line with how they genuinely experience their relationship with their body.

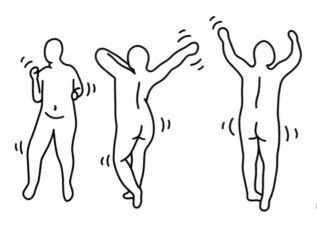

Are **problems** with sex common?

Like every part of our lives, experiencing problems with sex is very common. However, when it comes to sex, we often avoid talking to others and seeking help when things go wrong.

Sexual problems, or dysfunctions, include feeling pain during sex (see p.120), erection and arousal problems (see p.122), and issues with orgasm (see p.99). The *British Medical Journal* defines sexual dysfunction as a problem with sex that lasts for six months or more. However, problems can also be transient, and many who don't meet this criteria experience distress about an aspect of their sex lives that impacts their life and wellbeing.

Our sexual functioning can be affected by a huge range of factors. These include our mental and physical health; lifestyle choices; our stage of life; medication; injury; relationship quality; previous trauma; and distractions. For those with gender dysphoria (see p.19) or who are transitioning (see p.82), sexual arousal may feel challenging when their genitals feel incongruent with their gender. Dysfunction can also be situational. For example, situational-acquired erectile dysfunction can start after a period of normal sexual functioning and occur only when a partner is present. Other problems impact sex generally. For instance, low testosterone levels can reduce interest in sex, as can low oestrogen levels during breastfeeding, perimenopause, and menopause. Low oestrogen is also linked to vaginal dryness, which can make sex painful and affect our interest in sex. It's common for people struggling with a problem to feel a corresponding lack of motivation for sex, which compounds issues.

Our sexual functioning can also vary day to day. As with any activity, some days we feel strong, energized, and positive, other times we feel unmotivated or distracted. However, as sex is so meaning-laden, we often take any disruption to sexual function personally and

The way we manage issues can dramatically change the outcome.

many feel as though they're the only one struggling, leading to feelings of shame (see p.32). In turn, worry can imbed anxiety into our sex lives and interrupt our ability to focus on arousal. This can cause a transient issue to quickly become a persistent problem.

Seeking help

It can be incredibly challenging to reach out for help with our sex lives. For some, shame and embarrassment makes speaking even to a medical professional a challenge. We may feel that a problem will sort itself out and repeat experiences to see if things resolve. However, this doesn't address any changes we need to make – in our context, thinking, or physical involvement with sex. In fact, there's a great deal that can be done to overcome challenges. For example, medications along with psychological support can address some erection issues; practical measures such as lubricant can support physical problems such as vaginal dryness; and psychological hurdles around shame or questions of confidence can be tackled.

SEXUAL DYSFUNCTION

The UK Natsal-3 study, carried out 2010–2012 on over 15,000 men and women aged 16–74, showed that over half of women and almost half of men had encountered a sexual problem over the past year.

- 42 per cent of men who had sex in the past year experienced sexual difficulties.
- 10 per cent of men said that they were distressed or worried about their sex life.
- 51 per cent of women who had sex in the past year experienced sexual difficulties.
- 11 per cent of women were distressed or worried about their sex life.

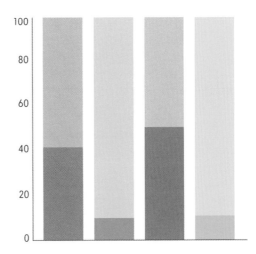

Is painful sex
normal?

No. Sex for people with all types of bodies can be painful for a variety of reasons. Pain is the body's way of telling us that something is wrong and is not something you should endure.

Vaginal pain

Vaginismus is the involuntary tightening of the vaginal muscles when penetration is attempted. It's thought to affect 1 in 500 people with vulvas, but cases are highly likely to be under-reported. Some experience it just with intercourse; others struggle with tampon use, medical checks, and solo and partnered activities, for example with finger or sex toy insertion. Penetration can be very painful, or impossible; descriptions of the pain felt vary, but it's often described as a burning or stinging sensation.

There are many reasons for vaginismus. It may arise where experiences such as urinary tract and sexually transmitted infections – or STIs (see p.204), medical procedures, and sexual trauma or assault, have linked pain to sex. Often described as psychosomatic, this doesn't mean it's not linked to physical factors. In all cases, the biological response is very real. The muscle tension is a response to the perception of a threat, with the amygdala, the brain's threat detector, likely playing a role.

Psychosexual therapy can be one source of support. A practical, and often successful, physical treatment is the use of dilators – tube-shaped devices that gradually increase in size, to help you become physically and emotionally comfortable with having something inside the vagina. These should be used under professional guidance and with a good-quality water-based lubricant for comfort. Many combine dilator use with clitoral stimulation, helping build an association between the genitals and pleasure, while arousal helps achieve comfortable penetration.

Pain in the vagina can also be a symptom of an STI or a common thrush infection. Other causes include an allergy to latex condoms; vaginal atrophy in menopause due to low oestrogen (see p.234); and bladder infections. Pain deeper in the pelvis can also make sex painful. This can be caused by conditions such as endometriosis – where tissue similar to the womb lining grows outside of the womb – and fibroids, both of which can require medical help.

For trans women, transfem or non-binary people who've surgically transitioned, the vaginal canal may not lubricate, which can cause friction and discomfort, so a good-quality water-based lubricant is important during penetration.

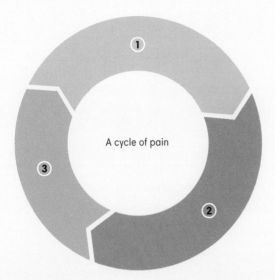

A cycle of pain

Painful sex can result from a combination of psychological responses and physical symptoms, creating a negative loop. Recognizing this can help you make adjustments to break the cycle.

- Repeated pattern of pain and avoidance can lead to recognition of a problem and a desire to seek help to address it.
- Seeking advice can help identify the cause and lead to solutions. This may include counselling, physical help from dilators where appropriate, lubricant, or sometimes medication or surgery. For conditions such as endometriosis, a programme of measures to ease pain during sex may be discussed.

1 When pain has been experienced during sex or a procedure linked with a sexual part of the body, the brain may anticipate pain at the next sexual encounter.

2 Expecting pain, the body activates a stress rather than arousal response. Physically, this can cause problems such as muscle tightness, leading to repeated episodes of painful sex.

3 If we don't change anything or seek help, painful experiences can be repeated. Sex and intimacy may be avoided and desire may drop.

Vulvodynia

This is persistent and unexplained pain in the vulva when the vulva appears normal and there's no other explanation for the pain. For some, it's described as being provoked as the pain flares up when the area is touched; or pain may be more constant in nature. It can impact people's sex lives and their daily functioning as it can mean that even simple activities such as sitting are painful.

Penile and testicle pain

People with penises can experience discomfort and pain from thrush and STIs, with chlamydia and other infections associated with swollen and sore testicles. A tight foreskin can also make sex painful as increased blood flow to the penis during arousal causes the penis to become swollen and tighter. Other conditions that can cause penile pain include prostatitis – inflammation of the prostate gland; and Peyronie's disease – a build up of fibrous scar tissue on the penis that can cause hard plaques to form under the skin. All of these conditions require medical attention.

Can erection issues be resolved?

There are a number of physical and psychological causes for erection difficulties. Often, with the right support and/or treatment, problems can be managed or overcome.

Physical causes of erectile dysfunction – whether someone is struggling to gain an erection or maintain one – include low testosterone, hypertension and cardiovascular issues, and diabetes, which can all impact erection quality. Spinal cord injury (SCI) is associated with erectile dysfunction as, dependent on the severity and location of the injury, it can disrupt the connection between the genitals and the brain. Some with SCI may still be able to have reflexogenic erections – ones that result from direct stimulation (see p.94) – sometimes with the help of specially designed devices. This may be possible if the nerve pathways in the S2–S4 sacral area that control the ability to have a reflex reaction are left undamaged. Erectile dysfunction can also be caused by a venous leak, which can lead to problems holding blood in the penis to maintain an erection.

Psychological erectile dysfunction counts for a large number of erectile dysfunction cases, particularly in younger men. Anxiety, depression, stress, and relationship problems can all interfere with the brain's role in the arousal process.

SEXUAL FUNCTION

A 2020 US study found that three in five men have had erectile dysfunction (ED) at some point. Increased age was a risk factor, though the gap between older and younger men wasn't significant.

- 56 per cent of 18–34 year olds affected.
- 63 per cent of over 55s affected.

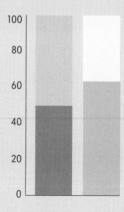

With the right interventions, erectile dysfunction can be successfully resolved for many.

Medical options

Medications and medical procedures require prescriptions and medical supervision.

- **Oral medications** called PDE5 inhibitors, such as Viagra or Cialis, can help improve erection quality by enhancing the effects of nitric oxide – the naturally occurring chemical that relaxes muscles in the penis (see p.94). These can help erections happen in response to sexual stimulation and arousal.
- **A vasodilator medication**, usually Alprostadil, can be given to help blood flow. This is administered via self-injection – with medical guidance – into the base or side of the penis shortly before sex, or a urethral suppository.

Non-medical options

- **A cock ring** is an easy and accessible option for those struggling to maintain an erection. Worn firmly, but not too tightly, around the penis base, it uses simple physics to trap blood in the penis shaft for a short time to maintain an erection. It can be especially helpful with conditions such as a venous leak or where medication may not be an option. Practising

putting one on alone, before sex with a partner, can build confidence using one. Rings come with a drawstring option or in a ring style and stretchy material is best. It's important to use the right size as when the penis expands, the ring needs to be removed quickly and easily. Rings shouldn't be left on for longer than 20 minutes and should be removed if there's numbing, discomfort, or pain to avoid damage. Some incorporate vibrators for extra pleasure and to stimulate partners.
- **A penis pump** – or vacuum erection device – is a hollow tube with a hand-powered or battery-powered pump. Placed over the penis, the pump sucks air out of the tube, creating a vacuum to pull the blood into the penis. Typically this is used with a cock ring.
- **Psychosexual therapy or counselling**, on its own or combined with medications or other methods, can help navigate the emotions and thoughts that can affect erections. Working through psychological hurdles and practising techniques at home that enable you to feel familiar with your body can help you return to a place of greater satisfaction with your sexual functioning.

How does **lifestyle** improve sex?

Our lifestyle – what we do and what we put in our bodies – forms part of the context of our sex lives, both directly and indirectly, affecting how we think and feel about ourselves.

Lifestyle factors, such as stress, sleep, diet, exercise, how much alcohol we drink, and whether we smoke, are often interrelated. For example, when we're stressed, we may struggle to sleep, or use food or alcohol as a coping mechanism. These coping techniques can affect our weight, self-image, and body confidence, and in turn impact our sex lives.

Does keeping fit improve sex?
Exercise influences how we feel physically and psychologically and can improve sleep, all of which can benefit sex. Regular moderate exercise keeps us supple and helps circulation, boosting genital blood flow to help facilitate arousal. For people assigned male at birth or others taking testoserone, exercise that helps reduce stomach fat may be helpful, as higher levels of fat here are linked to lower testosterone, which can dampen libido.

Sex itself can be seen as a mini workout. The activity increases the heart rate and uses muscles; while the physical tiredness felt after sex, combined with the release of feel-good neurochemicals, helps us relax and promotes sound sleep, benefiting health and wellbeing.

What about alcohol and smoking?
Alcohol can make us feel relaxed and less socially inhibited, which may have some benefits for consensual sex. However, it can also have a desensitizing effect on the body, and some feel less sensation during sex when they've been drinking, affecting their ability to orgasm. If someone is incapacitated from drinking, they can't legally give consent.

Smoking tobacco can negatively impact our circulation and in turn can contribute to sexual dysfunction if blood flow to the genitals is compromised.

Our wellbeing can influence the sex we're having, and sex can influence our wellbeing.

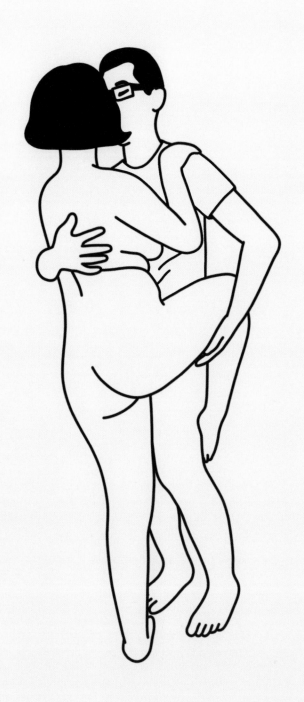

Attraction and desire

Why and how we experience attraction and sexual desire is a fundamental part of our understanding about sex. Some of the most commonly asked questions about sex are about how desire works – and how it can go from being instant and often overwhelming when we first meet someone, to waning over time, despite the original attraction still being there. Exploring the science behind desire – what can turn it on and off and how we can influence it – provides a crucial insight into what motivates us to have sex and offers invaluable tools to help us navigate our sexual lives.

Why does lust feel so intense?

The mixture of nerves, anticipation, and excitement that takes over when we're around someone we're attracted to is a feeling familiar to many, but what's actually going on?

In the early stages of attraction and lust, we can feel as though we're temporarily losing control. We may struggle to articulate ourselves, clam up, become unaccountably clumsy, and blush embarrassingly. Research from world-leading anthropologist, Dr Helen Fisher, reveals what's going on in our bodies when we feel lust and attraction, and how these two states can be the precursor to attachment, or romantic love. While there are no clearly set boundaries between lust, attraction, and attachment, each state has different, but interrelated, neurochemical characteristics that lead to recognizable behavioural changes. These different states are described as emotion–motivation systems.

Overcome by lust

Lust is a purely sexual state, arising when we feel an overwhelming physical attraction to someone and a desire for sexual gratification. It's driven by our sex hormones, with testosterone pushing the motivation for sex in people of all genders. For those who menstruate, oestrogen is also key, with many women reporting that they feel more sexually motivated around the time of ovulation, when oestrogen levels are at their highest.

THE FLIP SIDE OF ATTRACTION

When we feel pulled – physically, emotionally, and socially – to be with someone, the complex processes in our bodies and minds can make us feel as though we're not acting like ourselves. We may lean into performance-based behaviour – being the person we think someone will like rather than our authentic selves – which in turn makes our fear of rejection stronger.

A heady attraction

Closely related to lust, attraction is about selecting a partner. When we feel a strong attraction to someone, the neurotransmitters dopamine and noradrenaline come into play, creating a huge sense of excitement and anticipation that can see our appetite plummet and sleep go awry. The release of dopamine activates the brain's reward pathways (see p.56), driving us to seek

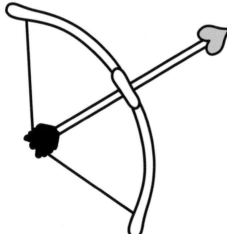

pleasurable activities and invest in what makes us feel good. Alongside this, noradrenaline leads to the release of adrenaline, leading to that familiar jittery, nervous state. To add to this chemical cocktail, a substance called phenylethylamine (PEA) is released, which plays a critical role in passionate love. PEA is thought to function like a natural amphetamine, which may be why the newly smitten sometimes describe feeling "high". Its effects are thought to fade over time – with feelings of infatuation usually receding by around 12 months. While we may mourn the loss of such intense emotions, this actually allows the body a much-needed break from its unsustainable state of high arousal.

Forming a bond

Building an attachment is critical for maintaining long-term relationships. Sex and touch release the chemicals oxytocin, commonly called "the love (or cuddle) hormone", and vasopressin, both of which promote bonding and attachment. These hormones also play a role in non-romantic and asexual relationships, too.

Why does lust feel so intense?   **129**

What happens when we feel desire?

Desire is interlinked with arousal but is a separate process. Desire is the motivation to be sexual; arousal describes the physiological and psychological processes that prepare us for sex.

In 2001, sexologist Dr Rosemary Basson developed a circular model of the sexual response process. This moved away from Masters and Johnson's linear model (see p.92) to integrate desire, emotional intimacy, and sexual stimuli as mediators of arousal. Her model focused on the female response but has relevance for all genders. She explained how desire is either spontaneous or responsive.

Feeling spontaneous sexual desire

Spontaneous desire describes the desire to be sexual that emerges seemingly out of nowhere and can result in physical signs of arousal (see 93). It can happen with little sexual stimulation or encouragement. Usually, though, something has initiated the response, even if we aren't aware of it; for example, the feel of a sensual texture on our skin, or catching the eye of an attractive stranger. This type of desire response is often experienced at the start of relationships, but usually doesn't endure constantly. Spontaneous desire is over-represented in the media, which is why many would likely define desire in this way.

Understanding responsive desire

Responsive desire arises, or is triggered, in response to stimulation, so isn't always there at the start of a sexual experience. This explains the phenomenon of not feeling in the mood for sex, but then really enjoying it once a sexual experience is underway. The feelings of desire come second to arousal, creating the desire to continue.

Understanding responsive desire offers us a huge amount of power and influence over our sex lives. We can appreciate how being receptive to the idea of a sexual experience with a partner, even if we don't feel motivated in that moment, can lead to a fulfilling experience. This can be helpful, for example, if a couple feels out of sync (see p.136) or someone is worried about low libido. For many in relationships, responsive desire becomes the main type of desire as familiarity can reduce spontaneity. Some also find responsive desire is their norm at the start of a relationship. This doesn't mean that something is missing, but rather that for them, desire emerges primarily in response to stimuli rather than in anticipation.

Satisfying physical and/or emotional experiences can increase motivation and openness to similar future events.

Initiation of sexual or sensual stimulation, such as partnered touch or kissing.

With sexual concordance (see pp.160–161), arousal intensifies as desire builds.

THE PROCESS OF RESPONSIVE DESIRE
This circular diagram, inspired by Basson's model of the sexual response process, illustrates how desire can occur after, and in response to, sexual arousal – so motivation for sex can happen after a sexual act starts.

If it's felt that conditions are conducive to sex, the body and mind may start to respond to the sexual stimuli.

Noticing signs of arousal can add to responsive desire. This comes after arousal and can increase motivation for sex.

Signs of physical arousal can occur, such as the start of an erection or vaginal wetness.

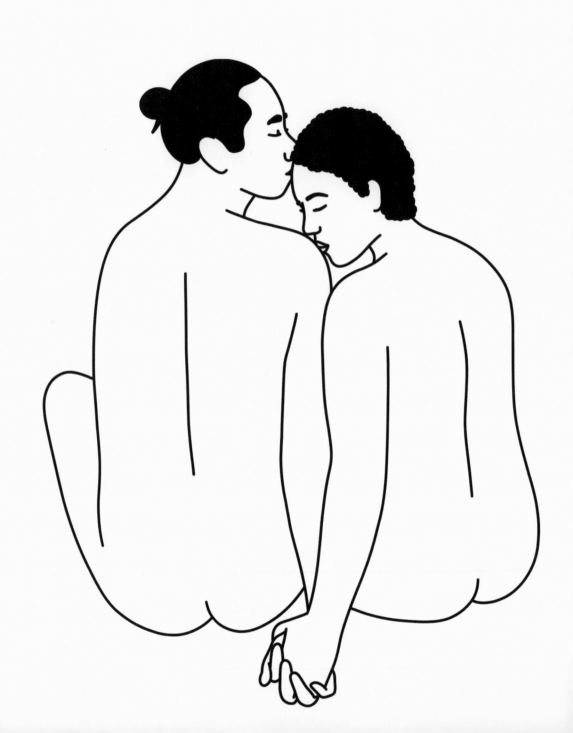

What are
pheromones?

These chemicals are produced by our bodies, but unlike hormones, pheromones are molecules that are expressed outside of the body – and some believe they play a role in desire.

Our senses are the gateway to how we experience the world and are crucial to our survival. Our noses contain sensory neurons; once a smell is detected, these send a signal to the olfactory bulbs in the brain's limbic system – the primitive part of the brain linked to instinctive behaviour. This is why smells can be so evocative and associated with certain times or people.

In the animal kingdom, pheromones produce scents that play a role in reproduction and survival. For example, species-specific pheromones produced by moths are thought to elicit arousal responses to help potential mates seek each other out. Observing the role of pheromones in animals has led us to seek parallels in humans, linking pheromones to attraction. However, the evidence that pheromones work in the same way for us is weak. Some studies have taken a component of male sweat and examined its effect on women. Dabbed on the upper lip of participants, it was found to produce a positive mood, however, the evidence was inconclusive.

As a species, we're a complex interaction of mind, body, and cultural influences. While changing one element of our biology might produce an effect, it can't control all the other variables that can account for why one person is more – or less – attracted to another person.

THE "McCLINTOCK" EFFECT

In 1971, there was much excitement about a study by biologist Martha McClintock looking at how cohabiting students' menstrual cycles synced over time. This was seen as evidence of the action of pheromones in humans. However, no research since has replicated or backed up her results.

Do aphrodisiacs work?

Ordering oysters in a restaurant is guaranteed to elicit at least one sexual innuendo, but is there any hard science behind our long-held belief in the aphrodisiacal powers of certain foods?

Throughout history, foods have been talked about as having aphrodisiac qualities, their potency holding the ability to boost levels of sexual arousal and desire. Despite this, disappointingly, there's no standup scientific evidence to prove these claims – if this was the case, the foods in question would probably be extortionately priced and in high demand. However, some foods do boast qualities and carry associations that are supportive of our sex lives and experiences of pleasure.

"Sexy" nutrients

The nutritional elements of some foods have antioxidant and anti-inflammatory qualities. Antioxidants contribute to improved circulation and relaxed blood vessels, which in turn play a key role in arousal by supplying blood to the genitals – an essential part of preparing the body for sex. Bright fruit and vegetables, pulses, seafood, and even dark chocolate, are all brimming with antioxidants.

Food can also make us feel good, and some of this is down to its composition and qualities. The perfect example is chocolate, which has sensual properties as it melts at slightly below body temperature. It's also linked to the production of the chemical serotonin –

A SEXUAL APERITIF

Many people feel turned off from sex after a big meal because of the unsexy sensation of feeling full and heavy, often accompanied by feelings of drowsiness as our bodies focus on digestion. If this is the case, don't feel afraid to mix things up and set eating aside for some pre-dinner sex.

chocolate contains small quantities of the amino acid tryptophan, a precursor to the neurotransmitter serotonin, which is linked to feelings of satisfaction and happiness.

Engaging the senses

Eating is a multi-sensory experience that can be sensual, emotive, and erotic and is often associated with intimacy. A meal is the start of many first dates, and people incorporate food into flirting and sexual play. A dinner with someone we like can increase attraction and build anticipation – evidence for the fact that desire doesn't happen in a vacuum but is always context dependent (see p.158).

All in the mind?

How we think and feel can be the mediator between food and sex, even if this is just a placebo. While not fully understood, it's thought that the power of suggestion can shape experiences. In one study, researchers studying brain scans found many opiate receptors activated by a placebo. In the context of sex, if we believe something is helpful, the act of giving it our attention puts desire in our mind, and the mere suggestion of sex can trigger arousal.

Food engages all the senses and can connect to evocative memories and associations.

Are we out of
sync?

We aren't perfectly matched and aligned with our partners in every single area of our lives, yet when it comes to our sex lives, we can feel that something is wrong if this isn't the case.

A "desire discrepancy" – not being motivated for sex at the same time as a partner – is far more common than being perfectly aligned sexually. However, often we're led to think of this as a problem of one partner having a low or high sex drive. This creates blame and leads us away from understanding that this isn't a problem if we know how to approach it.

Putting desire in context

Context plays a pivotal role in desire (see p.158), affecting how we feel and what's happening in our bodies (see opposite). We're often taught that desire is a constant and that changes are symptomatic of a bigger problem. In fact, anything happening around us has the potential to impact desire, so it can constantly fluctuate. For most, responsive desire (see p.130) is alive and well. If you find you're often out of sync with a partner, try the following:

• **Be open** to seeing where things go rather than focusing on an end goal, which can lead to worries about whether it will take too long to orgasm or that you're too tired.

• **Create context**. Change the mood by setting the scene and using cues to build sensuality and help align your focus.

• **Cue responsive desire in yourself**. Dip into your fantasies or engage your erotic imagination to help you lean into desire when with your partner.

• **Try not to make being out of sync a stress point** in your relationship. Feeling desire in response to physical stimulation rather than in anticipation of it is completely normal. However, making this a problem can create feelings of shame, which can then interrupt desire (see p.32).

A COMMON COMPLAINT

Up to 40 per cent of women aged 16–44 reported that lack of motivation for sex was impacting their sex lives.

How we feel can affect our physiological processes, helping explain desire discrepancies.

When we feel relaxed, levels of the stress hormone cortisol decrease.

When we feel stressed, circulating levels of the stress hormone cortisol are higher, which can also lead to a decrease in the sex hormone testosterone.

We can feel more alert, active, and relaxed and so may be more emotionally open and likely to lean into desire.

We may feel more fatigued and anxious, which in turn can dampen desire and motivation for sex.

Different experiences can lead partners to worry that they're sexually incompatible. Alternatively, acknowledging each other's feelings can promote understanding and motivate partners to navigate around perceived problems.

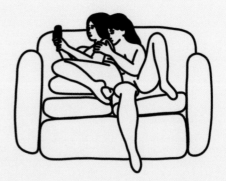

Does flirting improve sex?

Many animals engage in eye-catching flirting behaviours to signal their attraction to a potential mate. In humans, enjoying flirting can be a real boost to our sex lives.

When we flirt with someone – whether we increase our eye contact, change our body language, or engage in playful, suggestive behaviour – we communicate our attraction to them in a bid to get their attention.

The effects of flirting

Flirting, when welcome, can offer us a feel-good boost with knock-on benefits for our sex lives. For example, a flirty message sent to or received from a partner, or potential partner, during the day creates a sense of anticipation, bringing what we would like to do with them to the front of our mind. Anticipation is one of the body's natural aphrodisiacs. We get a release of the reward neurochemical dopamine (see p.56) when we expect good things to happen, as well as a rush of adrenaline that increases feelings of excitement and arousal. Flirting therefore preps us for arousal by building anticipation and creating feelings of desire.

Flirting also lets us know that we are wanted. When this is made obvious, it can boost our confidence and we may respond to a partner in a similar way. In long-term relationships, flirting can provide light relief, distracting us from the routines of daily life and reminding us what we first found so attractive about each other.

Eye contact and desire

Holding each other's gaze – a key component of flirting – can be especially arousing. When we gaze at a partner, this triggers the release of oxytocin, chemically connecting you to each other. Eye contact exercises

---

SEXUAL CURRENCY

This communication tool used in relationships has some overlap with flirting. Sexual currency is made up of non-sexual acts – such as extended hugs, prolonged eye contact, affirming compliments, playful touch, flirting, and suggestive messages – that we only do with a partner and which help keep a sexual connection alive (see p.220). This maintains a level of closeness outside of sex, nurturing erotic connections and fuelling desire.

are often used in couples' therapy as they help partners feel that they have each other's undivided attention. Psychologically, this attention and the feeling of being seen can be erotic, helping people to feel they're desired, in itself a turn on.

When flirting isn't welcome

While mutual flirting can boost desire or change the dynamic of a platonic relationship, it's important to check that flirting is reciprocal, as unwelcome flirting can be a big turn off and make some feel uncomfortable. Some may also find the direct nature of flirting too confronting, especially if other forms of communication are challenging. In this case, connecting with someone by finding common ground via shared interests and passions can be a more comfortable way to engage with someone we like.

TWO-WAY GAZE

One 2019 study looked at the link between eye contact and arousal, measuring changes to the skin. When couples made eye-to-eye contact, arousal signs increased, but dropped when they wore sunglasses, suggesting the interplay between sending and receiving eye contact was a key part of arousal.

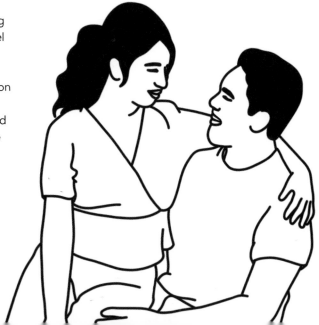

Can **novelty** kindle desire?

As humans, we habituate – our reaction to experiences that once caused a strong response can wane as they become familiar (see p.63).

The start of a liaison or relationship is a time of excitement, curiosity, and novelty. We explore each other emotionally and physically, desire is strong, and sex is likely to be more frequent. At this time we show our interest often through words and actions, known as sexual currency (see p.220), which acts as a motivator for sex.

However, the more time we spend with a partner, or partners, the less investment we tend to make. This behaviour mirrors observations in the animal kingdom, where mammals, especially males, become less intimate with a specific partner over time.

New horizons

To counter the tendency for desire to drop off, it's helpful to remind ourselves that a relationship is an active agreement – an ongoing work in progress that we need to invest in and nurture. Research has shown that how we spend time with a partner outside of the bedroom matters. When we share novel, interesting, and connecting non-sexual experiences with an intimate partner, this can increase the likelihood of feeling sexual desire, and as a result can lead to more sexual experiences. Novelty gives us a neurochemical dopamine boost (see p.56), which in turn encourages reward-seeking behaviours such as sex. Anecdotally, many people also report increased attraction to a partner when they see them anew through the eyes of others – for example, watching a partner give a speech at someone's wedding. Separating our partner from the view we have of them in our daily life can be a real boost to desire.

Not only can taking time to explore new interests and activities help our sexual relationship with a partner, but when we try new things we also learn more about ourselves. We expand our perspectives and move beyond our comfort zones; the corresponding satisfaction we feel from learning something new offers a boost to our self-confidence and self-esteem that can also benefit our sexual lives.

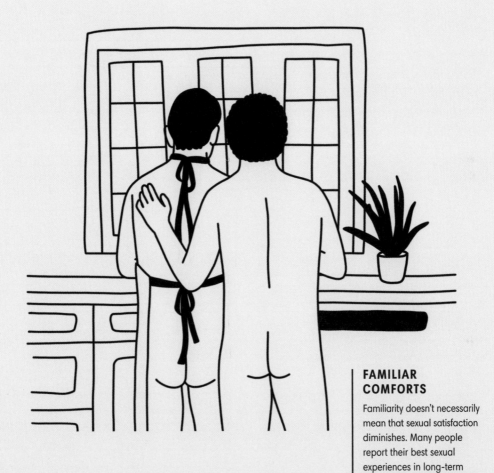

FAMILIAR COMFORTS

Familiarity doesn't necessarily mean that sexual satisfaction diminishes. Many people report their best sexual experiences in long-term relationships, when a partner knows their body well, they feel loved, and are with someone they feel relaxed and confident around.

What's behind human connection?

There's no exact science determining what sparks a connection between two people. Instead, the alchemy that brings partners together is dependent on a whole range of interweaving factors.

While there are biological drivers that motivate us to connect sexually and which play a key role in attraction (see p.128), physical and emotional elements of partnerships can fluctuate depending on what's going on in our lives. How we connect with another person sexually is an interplay of our genetics, life experiences, emotions, brain reactions, context, and personal psychology. All these elements are at play the moment potential partners meet, affecting whether a connection is made.

Our motivations

We know that some people are more sexually motivated and for them a physical connection is a primary driver for sex. How they personalize their desire can encourage or lessen the

Emotional intimacy
A strong emotional connection can help intensify a sexual one. When partners feel able to share feelings and desires, this can increase confidence and trust and help them explore each other and express themselves sexually.

High levels of emotional closeness can lead to great sex, and great sex can lead to feeling more emotionally intimate.

Physical intimacy
While physical intimacy is enough for some, it can lead to increased emotional intimacy. For example, where physical intimacy is strong, this can create vulnerability and an openness that can strengthen emotional connections.

A TWO-WAY STREET

Research supports thinking that sexual and emotional intimacy are interlinked. In 2016, two studies found that those with high sexual satisfaction had more sex, with more variety. Critically, an emotional connection meant they were able to communicate about sex.

potential for an emotional connection. Many also use sex as an initial way of exploring a partner; or they may wish to connect sexually without wanting an emotional connection.

For others, attraction starts with a sense of emotional closeness, which allows them to feel safe and open to exploring sexually. For demisexual people (see p.37), an emotional engagement is critical for sexual attraction to occur. For asexual people (see p.36), sex isn't a part of a connection, but they can enjoy emotional intimacy and close relationships.

In evolutionary terms, feeling safe promotes a desire for sex as it is non-essential when in survival and stress mode – for example, when dealing with the threat of an approaching predator. As we've evolved and adapted, this

feeling of safety has become not just physical, but also emotional – with sexual challenges often arising when there's emotional disruption.

A question of trust

The longer we spend with a partner, the more trust plays a role. Trust is a high-value principle in relationships and breeds emotional intimacy. Based on compassion, honesty, and consistency, trust promotes exploration and independence, known as the "dependency paradox". So, rather than becoming more dependent, we feel confident to explore. The emotional intimacy this brings comprises vulnerability, communication, and honesty. When we can express our needs to a partner, this can deepen sexual connections, too.

What's behind human connection?   **143**

What's a fetish?

The focus of a fetish doesn't have to be sexual in nature, but it can offer that person their peak level of sexual desire, arousal, and gratification.

A fetish is when we experience sexual desire and arousal in response to a particular non-genital body part, item of clothing, object, or practice. If you have a sense of needing an object to be present for sex to feel satisfying, and that sex is lacking without it, you may have a fetish. In theory, anything can be a fetish – popular ones include feet, hands, provocative clothing, or practices such as consensual voyeurism or role play, to name just a few.

The science behind why fetishes develop isn't concrete. One idea is that they occur with association and positive reinforcement. So repeated or intense association between an object and pleasure strengthens the association and reinforces a fetish. However, there's no one explanation for fetishes and having a fetish is most likely to be down to a mix of genetic, biological, social, and experiential factors.

Partners often enjoy exploring fetishes together – physically or through fantasy – and many find that incorporating a fetish into their sex play can be a real turn on. There are also multiple platforms for connecting with like-minded people to explore a fetish sexually.

Alternatively, much pornography is fetish-focused and can be explored individually.

Fetishes exist in varying intensities. Some experience peak arousal when their fetish is present but may enjoy sex without it. For others, a fetish must be present for them to be aroused and have satisfying sex.

Kink or fetish?

Kinks and fetishes can overlap, but kinks can be described as an overall erotic or sexual orientation, rather than a need for a particular thing. For some, a kink is a preference, so the kink, or kinky behaviour, may or may not need to be present to enjoy sex. For others, a kink can be described as an erotic orientation that's key for arousal, for example, if someone is aroused only when enjoying BDSM (see p.146).

Like fetishes, kinks are typically seen as falling outside of the mainstream, although this is subjective, as one person's kink may be another's norm. Vanilla sex is seen as the opposite of kink; however, again this is subjective as for some, vanilla can be delicious, adaptable, and give them exactly what they want.

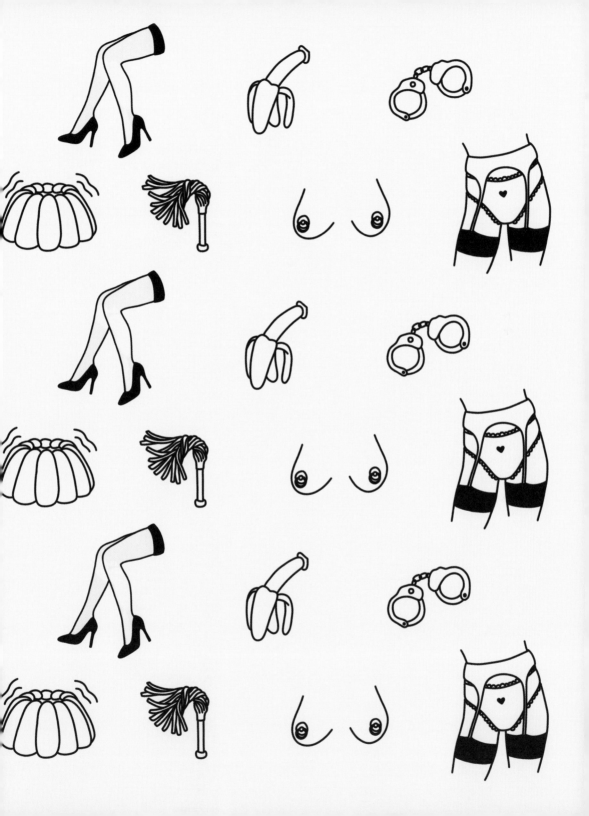

What's
BDSM about?

Bondage, discipline (or domination), sadism (or submission), masochism (BDSM) describes a consensual exchange of power, role play, and often intense sensory stimulation.

Like the rest of our sex lives, BDSM exists on a spectrum. A central theme of BDSM is power play, with partners in a dominant (dom) or submissive (sub) role, or switching. The power dynamic doesn't always involve sex, sometimes being acted out in everyday situations.

Bondage and discipline

Bondage is the practice of being physically restrained or tied up, or physically restraining a partner. Much of bondage is about giving up control to one partner, and the physical and psychological tension and anticipation created can be very pleasurable and erotic for all parties. Equipment such as bondage tape, cuffs, ties, or ropes can be used. Eye masks or blindfolds can add to the sensory experience and sense of giving up control.

Importantly, partners agree rules in advance. Discipline typically involves the dominant (dom) partner rectifying behaviour that could be considered to be rule-breaking and disciplining the submissive (sub) using physical or psychological cues.

Sadism and masochism

These are defined as taking sexual pleasure and enjoyment from experiencing physical or psychological pain (masochism) and inflicting pain (sadism). The pain can be created safely in various ways, for example, with hot and cold sensations, or with whips, flogging, or clamps, such as nipple clamps.

Safe practice

Clearly communicated consent, boundaries, and safety measures are essential to BDSM. Limits and expectations are agreed before roleplay begins. This is vital as BDSM can be intense, so knowing that it can be stopped at any time allows partners to let go and enjoy it fully.

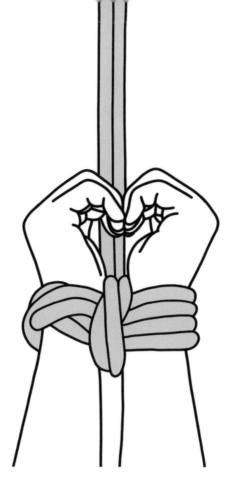

- Safe words for stopping should be clearly distinguishable from other words; for example, "no" might be misconstrued in BDSM so should be avoided. Many use a traffic light system. Green means someone is happy to continue; amber means things are beginning to feel intense and they're nearing their limit; and red means a limit is reached. If you use the word red, discuss in advance whether this means they should reduce intensity or stop completely.

- Agreeing limits is important. These allow the submissive partner to feel safe, while removing ambiguity for the dominant partner about what they can or can't do. "Hard limits" are absolutes, referring to things you don't consent to. "Soft limits" refer to consent given because the submissive partner may be interested, but unsure, and they want to see how they feel. Limits may change on different occasions, so it shouldn't be assumed that agreements previously made continue to be relevant.

What makes
holiday sex
so good?

A break from the norm and change of scene offers us a novelty-inspired neurochemical boost, but that's not all.

As well as activating the dopamine reward centre of our brains (see p.56), taking a break and enjoying new and enjoyable environments and activities has a whole stack of benefits that can give our sex lives a boost and help create, or reignite, those heady feelings of lust and attraction (see p.128).

Letting go of time

On holiday we can let go of time constraints and our preoccupation with to-do lists, work meetings, and everyday tasks. As we focus on the present, unencumbered by anxiety about where we need to be or what we need to do, this offers us the chance to enjoy sex that isn't limited to certain times of day or places; in turn, we're able to be more open to both spontaneous and responsive desire (see p.130) when they arise.

When holidaying with a partner, we naturally enjoy more quality time together, which can feel sparse in our normal lives. This can enhance our connection, which acts as a motivator

Being in holiday mode can mean we find it easier to switch off and feel turned on.

and increases our desire for each other. Even as parents on holiday with our children, being away from our everyday lives suggests relaxation and adventure, helping us reconnect with our partner and break away from our usual daily routines of parenthood.

A chance to recuperate

Being able to catch up on sleep is a holiday win that can also motivate desire. Getting enough sleep isn't just important emotionally and psychologically, but also biologically. When we're deprived of sleep, the body is more likely to produce the stress hormone cortisol, which can suppress our sex hormones. One study on women showed that sleeping

for one hour longer increased sexual desire the following day, with participants reporting a 14 per cent increase in partnered sex.

A sense of freedom

The disconnect from the rest of our lives, separation from any constraints we feel, and distance from those who know us can bring a sense of freedom to explore, experiment, and be curious. For those enjoying a holiday fling, a new environment can be intoxicating paired with the intensity we might feel when time with a new partner is limited; as a result we may feel freer to focus on what's happening in the here and now rather than where a liaison may be going.

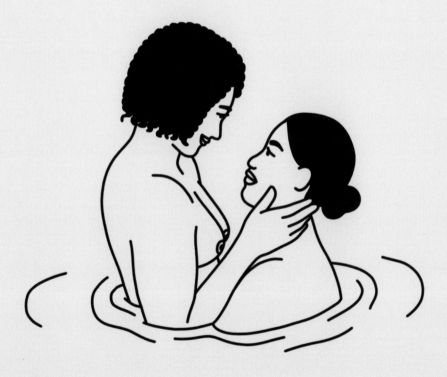

What's the best
time for sex?

While there are physiological processes that come into play here, our lifestyles and habits are likely to be bigger determinants than biology of how we manage our sex lives.

Given that the bulk of our sex lives happen in the bedroom, and most of us find ourselves there at bedtime, it's not a surprise that the majority of us have sex at night before we go to sleep.

However, despite bedtime being the most common time for sex, testosterone – one of our key sex hormones (see p.108), especially for men – surges in the morning. This suggests that without life constraints and the involvement of our consciousness – a major factor in desire – waking in the morning is when we would be most driven to act on feelings of arousal. Our own biological clocks – the body's natural circadian rhythms – that can influence whether we're night owls or early larks can also interact with hormones and play a part in when we are most likely to feel motivated to have sex.

As humans, we can't switch off our consciousness, which means that our reflective mind can override our biological drive. Likewise, our life set-up and circumstances play a big part in when we are likely to feel desire. So, if you're rushing to get ready for the day – and for some, also getting young children ready for their day – the busy and sometimes unpredictable nature of mornings makes sex first thing a challenge. For those with disabilities who may need to prepare and plan for sex, the spontaneity of sex in the morning is also unlikely to work.

What works for you

For some, the morning offers the chance to enjoy sex without the distraction of already being "in" their day, setting them up with a neurochemical boost at the outset. Others feel most relaxed at bedtime, when there's nothing to compete with sex aside from sleep, and the release of the neurochemicals associated with sex and orgasms – oxytocin, vasopressin, prolactin, and serotonin – can help to lull them to sleep.

Some people find sex after eating a turn off, disliking the feeling of physical pressure on their body when full, and are happy to sink into post-meal lethargy. For others, practicalities such as shift work can mean sex is only possible at certain times.

In reality, the best time of day to have sex is the time that feels right for you. Taking into account your preferences, lifestyle, and what makes you feel good psychologically can help you work out the times when you'll feel most motivated, receptive, and responsive to sex.

The best time for sex is when your preferences align with your lifestyle demands.

DAILY TESTOSTERONE LEVELS
Levels of this libido-driving hormone peak at 7–9am, then fall gradually during the day before rising again in the night.

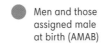 Men and those assigned male at birth (AMAB)

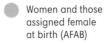 Women and those assigned female at birth (AFAB)

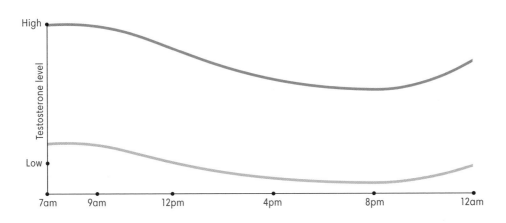

Are our
phones
in the way?

In many ways, our smartphones have become our primary relationships. We text more than we touch, and often gaze into our screens rather than each other's eyes.

Smartphones are attention thieves, which is exactly what they were designed to be. The access to information we get through smartphones has both helped and hindered our sex lives. The rise of available sexual content, on the one hand, has been an unreliable substitute for credible sex education; while also a gateway to exploring sexuality in lieu of more open conversations about sex.

A clear distraction
Although our phones are essential for connecting with others, when we're with someone, they do create a barrier, especially for non-verbal communication, which plays a critical part in our sex lives. In research conducted in 2020 by UK beauty brand *This Works*, over 25 per cent of people admitted that phones, laptops, and TV distracted them from intimacy. In the under 45s, using their phone was what most said they did in bed before sleeping, instead of reading, watching TV, cuddling, chatting, or having sex, despite the fact that 66 per cent said that the bedroom was where sex typically took place.

Being aware
When we're absorbed by our phones, we can miss bids for attention from partners, such as eye contact, verbal cues, or touch. These moments are fertile ground for triggering desire, so when we ignore them we are limiting our sexual potential.

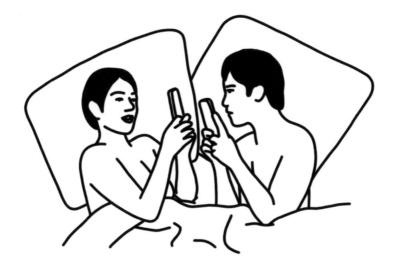

- Notice how often you reach for your phone and try to delay picking it up.
- Try tuning out from tech before bedtime. Aim to put your phone aside 30 minutes before bed and direct your attention to your immediate environment.
- Agree regular tech-free time with a partner, for instance, at mealtimes or when sitting talking on the sofa. Removing external demands anchors you in the moment, making connecting and leaning into pleasure more likely.

Unintentionally, our phones have become our permanent plus ones.

Can a sex break
reboot desire?

Taking a break from sex might not sound like a simple solution for boosting desire if it feels at a low ebb. However, a change of direction can sometimes be helpful.

Whether dips in desire are linked to anxiety around parts of the sexual experience, or there are differences in perceived levels of desire between partners (see p.136), pressing pause on a part of sex, rather than stopping sex altogether, can be enough to stop a problem escalating.

A different approach

Sexologists Masters and Johnson developed a technique called "sensate focus" in the 1970s to help those whose anxiety around penetration was affecting desire. The idea was to step back from penetrative sex for a period of time and work back to it in a managed way with a hierarchy of touch exercises, known as "in vivo exposure". This has been adapted in psychosexual therapy with some success, partly as it helps people to connect with pleasurable touch and their responsive desire.

However, it has also been criticized as an approach that isn't relevant for all groups, for example, for some who've experienced trauma who may find touch re-traumatizing. Importantly, there's no one-size-fits-all approach and the effectiveness of any technique can vary from person to person.

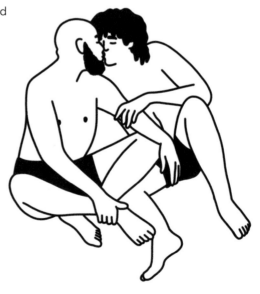

Exploring new routes

Masters and Johnson's basic premise can offer some helpful suggestions if you feel your sex life needs a reboot.

Removing, or avoiding, your primary way of being sexual together can encourage you to explore each other in different ways. This isn't just applicable to couples where intercourse is the dominant way of having sex, it's relevant for habituation around any type of sex. Often, many of our ideas around sex are socially conditioned, so creating alternatives helps us re-navigate our pleasure, which can flag up whether we're doing something out of habit or conscious choice. Refocusing on sensations alone, rather than where they might lead, can turn up the volume on our sensitivity. This encourages the release of dopamine from the brain's mesolimbic pathway (see p.56), which reinforces reward-related learning. In addition, for many, taking their main way of having sex away and being challenged to stick to these temporary rules is a turn on in itself. The build up of desire, wanting, teasing, and playful touch can heighten your sensitivity and leave you both feeling aroused, which in itself is a driver for more sex.

This isn't only applicable to partnered sex; this sensitizing technique can also be used for solo experiences, helping you explore new ways of reaching pleasure.

A FUN EXERCISE

If you're both game, a simple exercise can be a fun way to explore new paths to pleasure with your partner. Set a timer for 20 minutes. During this time, you are allowed to kiss, touch, and tease, but only the parts of the body that aren't normally associated with sex. Once the timer goes, you can either stop or carry on in whatever way you like, just focusing on what feels good.

Is make-up sex better?

For some couples, conflict can ignite desire and lead to passionate encounters, but whether or not this works for you is dependent on you and your relationship.

Conflict and disagreement are an expected part of relationships, as partnerships are made up of individuals simultaneously battling for dependence and independence. Whether make-up sex is more satisfying – or works as a method of relationship repair – is dependent on the level of resolution you and your partner manage to reach.

For those who feel happy that they can heal a rupture and put an argument behind them, sex can act as part of the reconciliation process. As you are both likely to be in an emotionally heightened state, this can charge the sexual experience and lead to more passionate and intense sex (see opposite).

Make-up sex can also act as a way of deepening intimacy. This is because conflict and disagreement – with the associated risk of losing a relationship – along with resolution, can increase our vulnerability; this in turn can make us feel closer as we work through problems together.

If you or a partner find it challenging to put an argument to bed or to find resolution, then make-up sex is unlikely to be a good solution. In this situation, we're prone to retreat into ourselves rather than moving towards each other and you will probably struggle to desire sex in the moments after conflict. Trying to summon up the desire to have sex when you don't want to is most likely to build feelings of resentment that can be damaging for your sex life and your overall mental health.

Importantly, make-up sex should always be mutual and consensual. If it becomes a pattern you rely on for sex, this probably isn't the most productive relationship dynamic and signals that you might need to find alternative ways to inject passion into your sex lives.

During conflict, the amygdala – the emotional centre of the brain – is activated, sending the brain into flight-or-fight mode.

In this state of high alert, the stress hormones adrenaline and cortisol are released. Emotions can feel heightened or out of our usual control.

Stress hormones also have a physiological effect on our bodies, increasing heart rate, temperature, and blood flow to prepare us for action.

This heightened state creates tension and passion.

A process called "arousal transfer" may happen, where you move from one heightened state to another. This can lead to make-up sex that may be exciting and passionate.

Alternatively, heightened tension can act as a desire brake (see p.158). Couples need to resolve any conflict before they can contemplate sex.

Passion and emotion are present in both love and conflict.

What turns us
On or Off?

Each person's motivation for sex is influenced by myriad factors that can inhibit or excite desire and, in turn, our degree of arousal – showing us there's no normal when it comes to sex.

In the 1990s, Erick Janssen and John Bancroft, sexologists from the Kinsey Institute – the research centre studying human sexuality – devised a concept known as "the dual control model of sexual response". This helped explain how desire could be turned on or off – excited or inhibited – by external factors, taking our understanding of arousal beyond the purely biological.

This sexual inhibition system (SIS) and sexual excitation system (SES) essentially sets out sexual responses as governed by a brake and accelerator, where the sensitivity of each pedal is person-dependent. There is much variability, as thoughts, attention, memories, context, and any stimulation balances inhibition and excitation. The system is governed by the brain, which constantly assesses the input it receives about what's going on around us. This, in turn, affects how we think and feel and whether or not it's a good, or appropriate, time to be aroused.

Putting desire in context

The duality of this model means that during arousal, like the brake and accelerator of a car, we're activating one pedal while we ease off the other. This can explain why someone may start to feel in the mood for sex, but when a partner touches a certain part of their body they feel instantly turned off as the touch activated their brake. Or someone may be more easily aroused in a certain context – for example, if flatmates or children aren't at home, this pushes their accelerator. It can help us understand why we might struggle to get going sexually, or feel neutral or ambivalent at the start of sex, as our mind processes events.

This award-winning scientific model is used around the world in sexuality research. It shows that while there are universal aspects of sexuality, functioning, and behaviours, we can't consider these without also taking into account the influence of a person's individual nature when thinking about our desire for sex.

Identifying accelerators and brakes

Understanding the dual control model shows us how knowing our sexual preferences can be so helpful for making sense of our sex lives, especially if we feel distressed by struggling to become aroused. Self-questioning can help you identify your own brakes and accelerators:

• Is there a part of your body that instantly makes you feel more interested in or open to the idea of sex when touched?
• Do you feel more relaxed in certain contexts, for example when the lights are switched on or off, or if music is playing?

• Are you very easily distracted by noises or what's going on around you during sex?
• Are you more easily turned on by a partner you're close to, or one you don't know well?
• Do you notice a change in how interested you are in sexual experiences, either with yourself or with a partner, dependent on how stressed or worried you are?

These questions may feel obvious, but all of these factors act as prompts that distract us from being in the moment. By paying attention and making changes to suit our preferences, we can start to ease off the brakes.

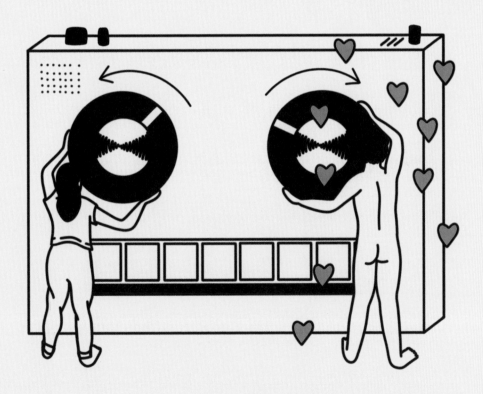

Why am I aroused when I don't feel desire?

Experiencing a disconnect between our subjective desire – how we're feeling emotionally or mentally – and our body's signs of physical and physiological arousal can be confusing.

Feeling that our body and mind aren't working together sexually is a very common experience, known as arousal non-concordance, a term popularized by Emily Nagoski in 2015 in her book *Come as You Are*. This can happen when our body shows signs of arousal yet we don't feel psychologically turned on; or conversely, we feel desire but our body isn't physically aroused.

Arousal non-concordance can happen in situations such as medical or hands-on examinations, where you might notice a physical response, such as increased lubrication or an erection, but are not thinking about sex. This is because the brain has coded what is happening as sexually relevant, for example, the sensation of touch, but you don't feel psychologically turned on or attracted to the person touching you. It's your body's involuntary and automatic physical response to touch. In terms of the dual control model discussed on pages 158–159, your brain has put the foot down on the accelerator.

This explains why some victims of sexual assault describe having experienced physiological responses that align with arousal, despite being in a situation that was traumatic, non-consensual, and where they had no subjective sexual desire. Their body responded physiologically in a way that was outside of their control. Past trauma can also cause the brain to translate sex as dangerous, painful, or threatening; this can make arousal challenging for some, even if they're in a current context where sex holds a more positive meaning.

This highlights the critical importance of communication when it comes to our sex lives – understanding that signs of arousal, such as vaginal wetness, are not consent if this hasn't been clearly communicated. Generally, our brain receives many sexually relevant signals from our environment and these are likely to outnumber the cues each person finds subjectively sexually arousing.

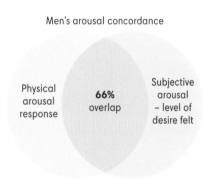

Women's arousal concordance

| Physical arousal response | **26%** overlap | Subjective arousal – level of desire felt |

Men's arousal concordance

| Physical arousal response | **66%** overlap | Subjective arousal – level of desire felt |

Slow to respond

Arousal non-concordance can also lead to confusion and upset if we are in a sexual situation where we do feel desire but are struggling to get our mind on our side, which hampers our physical arousal. For example, factors such as stress and distraction can disconnect us from arousal-concordance so we're not physically prepared for sex. Life stages such as menopause, where low oestrogen can cause vaginal dryness, can also mean that the sexual response in our bodies and minds may not align. If we don't understand what's happening, this can quickly turn to self-criticism or self-blame.

However, when we know our bodies, we can implement really important changes in our sex lives. For example, we can introduce lubricant, or direct our attention to sensations by using mindfulness-based techniques (see p.180) to better align our subjective arousal and our physical response.

SEXUAL ALIGNMENT IN MIND AND BODY

In a seminal study from 2010 led by psychologist Meredith Chivers, men had a higher correlation than women between their genital response and their psychological desire for sex. Men's sexual concordance was 66 per cent compared to 26 per cent in women. One possible reason is that as men's physical arousal is more obvious, this could help them connect more quickly with this and feel corresponding desire.

Can I be more aware of my arousal?

Noticing our bodies' signs of arousal is an important part of our sexual experience, as it's our perception of how aroused we are that gives arousal meaning, building our desire for sex in the moment.

Taking time to work out what you like and don't like can help you to focus on physical sensations and avoid self-judgment about whether your body is responding properly, which can often get in the way during sex.

Mapping our signs of arousal

The following exercise will help you build your relationship with your body and can be an ongoing and repeated practice. You can take the exercise as little or as far as you want in terms of pleasure – there's no goal, just the intention of erotically navigating and exploring your body and being aware of how arousal manifests for you and increases your desire.

- **Wearing whatever clothing**, underwear, or nakedness feels right for you, sit or lie somewhere comfortable, where you feel relaxed. Consider your conditions for good sex (see opposite) and lean into what helps you in terms of sensory cues, such as music, lighting, and temperature, to help you ease off your desire brake (see p.158).
- **Next, practise deep, controlled breathing** to settle into your body. This promotes relaxation by triggering the parasympathetic nervous system. Inhale for a count of four, hold the air in your lungs for a count of four, exhale for a count of four, then hold your lungs empty for a count of four before taking the next breath. Do this three or four times. Focus on the path of your breath as it travels into your nose and mouth, through your body, and back out. Be aware of which parts of your body move as you breathe and notice where you place your hands, how you're sitting or lying, and any sensations.
- **When you're ready**, take your hands to the top of your head and hold them there. As and when you desire, start to run your hands over your head and through your hair, then down your face, ears, and neck, using whatever pressure or style of touch you like. Be explorative and, importantly, use pleasure as your guide, checking in with feelings and thoughts, which tend to be the parts of ourselves that give or restrict permission.
- **As you take this touch down the body**, vary it – try trailing the fingertips over the skin, using the flat of your palm, or moving direction and motion. Don't avoid areas

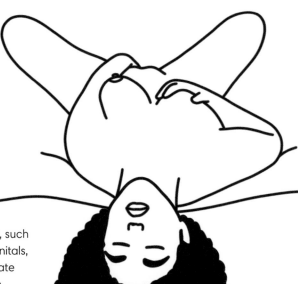

associated with sex, such as the breasts or genitals, but try not to separate them out – focus on journeying around from head to toe.

- **If you're feeling distracted**, consider why this might be happening when you're in a situation with no pressure or expectations. Is there an area or type of touch evoking that reaction? Which parts feel good, and which seem to take away your sexual charge? What's happening in your mind and emotions? Are you avoiding areas out of habit? When we map touch we can be aware of things that we might be doing unconsciously, often out of self-judgment about how our bodies look, feel, or function. Sometimes our self-image or shame can mean we don't allow ourselves to be fully in the moment. Recognizing this and focusing on sensations can help us to let go of negative messaging and experience pleasure fully.

WHAT WE NEED FOR GOOD SEX

There are certain conditions that help us to control our arousal concordance (see p.160) – aligning desire with physical arousal. In her book, *Mind the Gap*, Dr Karen Gurney points to three areas that facilitate good sex:

- Psychological arousal – feeling relaxed and turned on psychologically.
- Pleasure from physical touch.
- Being in the moment – without distraction.

In a perfect world, these would all be as close to our ideal as possible to maximize our pleasure. However, imbalance is likely, but recognizing their input helps us to influence our levels of desire and, if partnered, close a desire gap.

Does it matter who initiates sex?

Most couples build up routines around how sex typically starts – often using personalized codes or familiar language. However, where patterns become set, problems may follow.

In heterosexual relationships, gender norms around who initiates sex are well ingrained into many people's sexual scripts. Common assumptions are that men initiate and women respond, or that men think about sex more, so are naturally more likely to initiate it.

Narratives around testosterone fuel the idea that spontaneous desire (see p.130) is always dominant in people with penises than those with vulvas. However, these assumptions aren't facts and aren't applicable to everyone. Despite this, they can set up expectations and reinforce ideas about what sex should look like, even if that isn't working for us. Phrases such as, "If I don't initiate sex it will never happen", or "You only kiss or approach me when you want sex" are commonplace in conversations where sex has become a pressure point.

Exploring different roles

Looking at different relationship models throws up some interesting statistics and can encourage people to break out of assumed roles where these are unhelpful. In a 2018 survey of 4,175 people in the US, 28 per cent of heterosexual women said they often or always initiated sex compared to 50 of heterosexual men. However, in gay and bisexual couples, where couples are less likely to conform to gender norms, initiating sex is almost evenly split between partners.

Interestingly, where heterosexual women used fantasy in their sex lives, the numbers who initiated sex rose significantly, increasing by 25 per cent, suggesting that engaging in fantasies helps them to break free of expected gender roles.

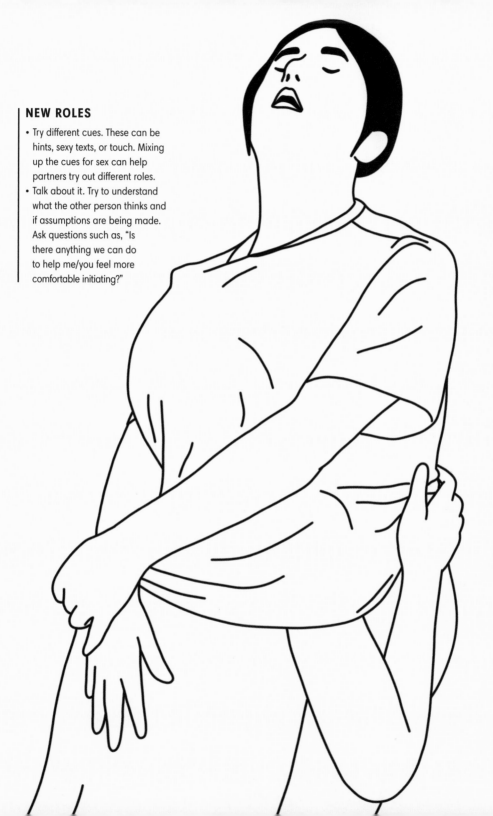

NEW ROLES

- Try different cues. These can be hints, sexy texts, or touch. Mixing up the cues for sex can help partners try out different roles.
- Talk about it. Try to understand what the other person thinks and if assumptions are being made. Ask questions such as, "Is there anything we can do to help me/you feel more comfortable initiating?"

How can I say no without a partner feeling rejected?

Often, worries about leading a partner on mean that we avoid intimacy – or anything that could potentially lead to sex – in an attempt to manage our partner's expectations.

Often, the absence of desire for sex means that we instinctively feel we're not in the mood. Whatever your reason for not wanting sex at a particular place, time, or moment, you always have the right to say no. Communication is critical in any scenario with a partner. Where there's mutual respect, finding a way to say no without making your partner feel rejected can enhance trust and understanding.

Interestingly, research has uncovered 237 reasons why humans have sex and, not surprisingly, motivation isn't always linked to desire (see p.42). While sex can be about wanting pleasure this isn't always the case; for example, it may be about wanting to feel close, or simply to help us sleep better. However, we sometimes find that our openness to a potential interaction leads to responsive desire and the subsequent enjoyment of a sexual encounter (see opposite and p.130).

A GENTLE LET-DOWN

- Avoid ambiguity. Not knowing where we stand is a breeding ground for overthinking. Be clear about what you're happy to do, for example, "I'm not in the mood for sex tonight, but I'd love to cuddle up and watch a movie in bed".
- Listen to their response so your partner feels heard. Phrases such as, "I understand why you feel like that but I'm not in the right headspace" will help your partner feel acknowledged.
- If you're open to trying something but want to see how it goes, communicate this. Feeling pressure to follow through can be a turn off, triggering the fight-or-flight stress response. Conversely, communicating how you feel can free you to focus on what's happening in the moment and may lead to responsive desire.
- Offer reassurance and love, clarifying that saying no on this occasion isn't saying no to them. Sex is a mutual experience and a part of relationships that needs constant negotiating.

COMMUNICATION = UNDERSTANDING

Learning to communicate our needs to a partner can ensure understanding, avoid hurt, and sometimes gives us the freedom to lean into responsive desire.

When we **communicate clearly that we don't want sex...**

When we fail to say **that we're not in the mood for sex...**

This reduces the worry that affection will send out the wrong message. We feel free to enjoy the intimate act of a cuddle without worrying about where this might lead.

We may turn away from bonding acts of affection, such as a cuddle, to avoid giving the wrong message.

Without explaining our feelings in the moment, our partner can feel rejected.

We may simply enjoy the physical intimacy, which also triggers the release of bonding oxytocin.

This physical intimacy may trigger responsive desire (see p.130). Our mood may change as we respond to the sensuality of the moment, and we may go on to enjoy sex with our partner.

Clear communication avoids a partner dwelling on a misinterpretation that could potentially damage trust.

Sex gaps

When it comes to sex, we often find ourselves facing gaps between our real-life experiences of sex and our perceived ideals. This is compounded by the fact that the versions of sex we so often see in the media are often not relatable. To complicate matters, we may turn to incorrect assumptions on sex to bridge these gaps, and treat our sexual thoughts and feelings as facts, leaving many of us stuck in unfulfilling sexual patterns. Being equipped with the right information can motivate us to move out of sexual comfort zones and help increase our sexual satisfaction.

Why does my partner orgasm **more?**

A discrepancy in orgasms between partners, commonly referred to as the "orgasm gap", does everyone a disservice.

Failing to orgasm can affect any of us. However, when it comes to orgasm rates between couples, the biggest gap occurs between heterosexual partners, where men consistently orgasm more than women. The orgasm gap was identified early in modern sexual research. The 1953 Kinsey Report, *Sexual Behaviour In The Human Female*, found that, prior to marriage, 36 per cent of women had never climaxed, while 100 per cent of men had. Further studies highlighted how, during sex with men, women consistently reported a lower orgasm rate than their partners. Research shows that this gap dramatically reduces, and sometimes almost disappears, when women masturbate or have same-sex experiences.

THE ORGASM GAP

A study in 2017 compared orgasm rates over a month in adults of different sexual orientations. Heterosexual women had the lowest rate. Women were more likely to orgasm if they received oral sex, manual clitoral stimulation, and deep kissing.

95 per cent of heterosexual men said they usually or always orgasmed when sexually intimate with a partner.

89 per cent of gay men usually or always orgasmed when sexually intimate with a partner.

A flawed narrative

Sexology psychologist, Dr Laurie Mintz, author of *Becoming Cliterate*, believes one of the key predictors of the orgasm gap is a lack of education around how female sexual pleasure works. Historically, the biological, social, and educational focus on penetrative vaginal intercourse can be seen as having elevated men's sexual pleasure over women's. By focusing on intercourse solely as sex, and using the terms interchangeably, insufficient attention has been paid to direct clitoral stimulation – the way most people with vulvas orgasm. A narrative has developed that it's trickier for people with vulvas to orgasm – despite the fact that in studies, a higher orgasm rate in lesbian and bisexual women shows that clitoral stimulation brings more frequent satisfaction. Implanting the belief that vulval pleasure is tricky can influence experiences, with less focus on pleasure and an idea that orgasms often aren't attainable. The expectation is that sex is often unsatisfying and orgasm a bonus.

Feeling a partner isn't experiencing pleasure fully can be frustrating for both. Getting to know our bodies and communicating about pleasure can help close this gap and create more satisfying sex for all.

Saying "vagina" instead of vulva ignores the clitoris, one of the key sources of pleasure.

88 per cent of lesbians usually or always orgasmed when sexually intimate with a partner.

66 per cent of bisexual women usually or always orgasmed when sexually intimate with a partner.

65 per cent of heterosexual women usually or always orgasmed when sexually intimate with a partner.

Does faking it
matter?

While faking an orgasm with a partner may feel harmless, it can have repercussions for our sex lives – the perceived short-term gain can have a long-term negative impact.

Faking orgasms during partnered sex isn't exclusive to heterosexual women, although statistics show that they're more likely to do this. One US study found 58 per cent of women had faked an orgasm; a separate study found 28 per cent of men had also faked an orgasm during penetrative vaginal sex.

Why do we fake orgasms?
The following reasons are commonly cited:

- **To protect a partner's feelings**. Women may be more inclined to feel responsible for how partners feel. In a 2022 US YouGov poll, 56 per cent said they were people pleasers compared to 42 per cent of men. Many continue faking as they worry confessing will break trust. Guilt builds, activating the amygdala – the brain's emotional centre – forming a hard-to-break pattern.

- **We assume that difficulties** reaching orgasm is a problem that lies with us. Self-criticism induces shame, which we internalize.
- **We don't want a partner to think we're "bad at sex"**, or for our failure to orgasm to influence how they feel about us.
- **To bring sex to a close**. Ingrained narratives tell us that an orgasm is the natural end to a successful sexual encounter.

However, these efforts are flawed. By prioritizing a partner's pleasure, we can end up expecting and receiving less ourselves, which dampens our motivation for sex. We also add to sexual myths, such as people with vulvas climaxing easily during penetrative sex. When a partner assumes they're satisfying us, they repeat sexual behaviours they think are working, but which don't bring genuine sexual pleasure.

Closing the orgasm gap

There are many rewards and benefits of sex, of which orgasm is just one. However, a major obstacle to reaching orgasm is our focus on achieving it. If climaxing is a challenge, consider the following:

- **Get in touch with what feels good**, bearing in mind this is subjective. Familiarizing yourself with your body then showing a partner what feels good should be fun and something to celebrate, rather than indicating a lack of sexual skill.
- **Clarify, don't assume**. Being curious, asking what a partner likes, and sharing what we enjoy can be empowering and lead to highly pleasurable partnered sex.
- **Stop chasing orgasm as a goal**. Sex can be extremely pleasurable without an orgasm, but if we focus on climaxing this

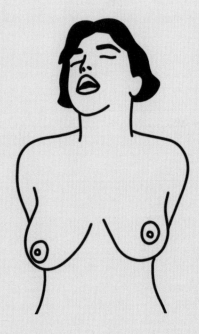

creates pressure. In some non-sexual situations, such as a work deadline, a little pressure may help us perform. However, with sex, pressure distracts us, redirecting our focus away from arousing sensations that can lead to an orgasm. Practices such as mindful or tantric sex (see p.180) focus on the experience of sex, rather than a desired result.

Why does onscreen sex look so exciting?

There's often a sizeable gap between our perception of the sex we're having and the sex we see on screen. However, onscreen depictions of sex are frequently misleading.

When good-quality sex education is lacking, many are left with questions when it comes to understanding the full nuances of sex. Even when conversations about sex are more open, curiosity is a huge driver and we may turn to sources such as onscreen sex and pornography for some extracurricular education.

However, sex in dramas and pornography isn't usually designed to be educational. As a consumer, we may logically know this, but it's still likely to influence our ideas about sex if other sources of information are missing. With porn especially, the widespread introduction of smartphones in 2007 transformed ease of access, particularly for younger viewers. Our education has struggled to provide a counter narrative to the skewered representations of sex on offer. Talking about "porn literacy" – the acceptance that many young people view porn – can help viewers at least think critically about what they view.

Far from reality

Onscreen depictions of sex often model a type of sex that looks good on camera, but doesn't necessarily replicate what feels good in person. The sex doesn't usually reflect the imperfections of real-life sex, making little allowance for unpredictable noises bodies can make, the discomfort of a position, or the distraction of getting a text.

Instead, the sex we watch in dramas or via pornography is nearly always spontaneous, with couples in the mood for sex at the same time; penetration appearing to be the best way to orgasm; and as soon as penetration starts, pleasure is instant, with couples climaxing simultaneously. In addition, sexual positions are frequently unrealistic and hard to achieve in real life, with penetration happening at awkward angles to look good on screen.

Mimicking or copying the onscreen sex we view is a common behaviour as it can make us feel as though we're armed with sexual knowledge or expertise; but the irony is that it regularly has the opposite effect. Working out what feels good as we go along is by far the best way to navigate a sexual experience.

A welcome change is the increased use of intimacy coordinators on some productions (see right). As well as creating less intimidating conditions for actors, by ensuring sex looks realistic the viewer stays focused on what they're watching, rather than being distracted by thoughts such as, "That's not what it's like for me!"

A positive outlook

The flipside to how we view pornography is that for some it offers a sense of inclusion and reassurance. For example, those who feel that their sexual desires aren't represented in the mainstream may find a community online and feel a sense of belonging (see p.60). It may also help some accept their sexuality and preferences and reduce feelings of shame. For those in isolated communities, the internet may offer a sense of connection.

INTIMACY COORDINATORS

A big advance in many onscreen dramas today is the introduction of intimacy coordinators. As well as guiding the choreography of sex scenes to make them more true to life, they check for consent and facilitate communication between actors and directors to keep actors safe.

Why does talking about sex feel taboo?

While there's been a huge shift in the conversation about sex in the past few decades, normalized references to sex still aren't embedded in our everyday language.

We often see those professionally associated with sex, or working within the sexual wellness or pleasure industry, considered as risqué, rather than positioned alongside other health professionals. Conversations about sex are assumed to be sexualized or sexualizing by nature, providing another reason for us to prefer to veer away from the topic of sex in society.

We also still hold strong the idea that talking about sex with children will sexualize them earlier, when in fact research shows that with better age-appropriate sex education (see p.24), adolescents had a more delayed sexual debut and used contraception. In one scheme in Mexico, where trained teachers taught sex education, 83 per cent of students used contraception, compared to 58 per cent where teachers were untrained. Numerous experts and sexuality professionals advise that age-appropriate sex education can emphasize the critical importance of consent and protect children from sexual violence in terms of identifying inappropriate touch or contact. Also, when information on sex isn't readily available, misinformation creeps in. For example, if teenagers aren't given comprehensive, accurate information, they may pay undue attention to inaccurate information from peers and online sources.

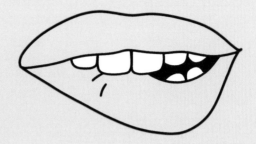

An awkward conversation

If we're talking to someone who is uncomfortable with the topic of sex, biologically and innately we can read their discomfort. The science of body language - kinesics - shows how non-verbal cues are part of our communication. We instantly pick up if there is an avoidance of eye contact or a shift in body language, such as crossing arms or putting a hand to the face - known as micronegative messages - that can signal discomfort, embarrassment, and shame. Or we may send out these signals when we internalize the culture of silence around sex.

Prioritizing sexual wellbeing

It makes sense that the number of people having sex is disproportionate to how much sex is talked about in an educational, destigmatizing, and non-shaming way. Of course, we shouldn't feel that we have to share information about our sex lives if we don't wish to - for some, a sense of privacy around sex is exactly what feels right. However, for others, the invisibility of sex in mainstream conversation creates a sense that it doesn't belong there.

A 2021 study by Peanut and Headspace, focused on women, highlights how this lack of conversation can have repercussions on sexual health and wellbeing. It found that only 27 per cent would talk to a doctor about their sex life, and that only 13 per cent talked to friends as a way to improve their sex life. Despite this, 70 per cent said they wanted better access to information that could improve their sex live.

Despite the predominance of sexual references in society, we often feel awkward talking about sex.

Why can sex feel like a performance?

A common concern about sex that people describe is feeling a sense of detachment – focusing on what they're doing rather than how they're feeling. The impact on pleasure is clear.

Sex is both doing and feeling. The mind-body connect is well evidenced when it comes to sex, showing we're unable to switch off our cognitive function during sex. Problems arise when self-critical and distracting thoughts interrupt physiological arousal processes (see p.92). The brain can be thought of as the biggest sex organ in the body so we need it on side during sex.

Intrusive thoughts

Sex can feel like a performance when we're preoccupied with our partner's experience, and how their perception of us measures how we're doing sexually. We may find sex peppered with thoughts on how we're "performing" and what we think we should be doing. Often, these thoughts come from embedded sexual scripts. For example, we may be thinking, "I hope I look okay from this angle" or, "I feel it's taking them too long, aren't I doing a good enough job?" or, "I really want to change position but I don't want to look like I'm not enjoying this."

Much of this comes from ideas we have about how sex *should* be (see p.52), often reinforced by the lack of diversity we see around sexual experiences in the media. Feeling as though we're performing is fuelled by the idea that sex is measurable in some way by the goals achieved, minimizing the idea of sex as a subjective experience.

Applying the brake

Feeling as though we're performing during sex creates stress, perceived by the body as a threat. The brain switches into its evolutionary fight-or-flight mode, triggering the release of cortisol and adrenaline, and blood flow is prioritized to areas such as the muscles and away from genitals, as arousal isn't critical at this point. The brake is pressed on desire (see p.158), interrupting arousal and, in turn, sex.

Intrusive thoughts can derail pleasure.

Spiralling away from pleasure

The irony is that these concerns take us away from the experience of sex. We start to pay less attention to physical cues and pleasurable sensations, which recede into the background as we give most attention to self-evaluating thoughts. The effect is like turning down the volume on physical sensations, making pleasure and satisfaction less likely. Ultimately, this dampens our overall desire for sex.

PERFORMANCE ANXIETY

This isn't the same as feeling that you're performing during sex, although it may arise from the cycle of negative thoughts that can end up interrupting desire and arousal. When worries about our ability to experience sexual desire and arousal creep in, this may lead to sexual dysfunction (see pp.118–123). A cycle can ensue, as anticipation about future events creates further anxiety.

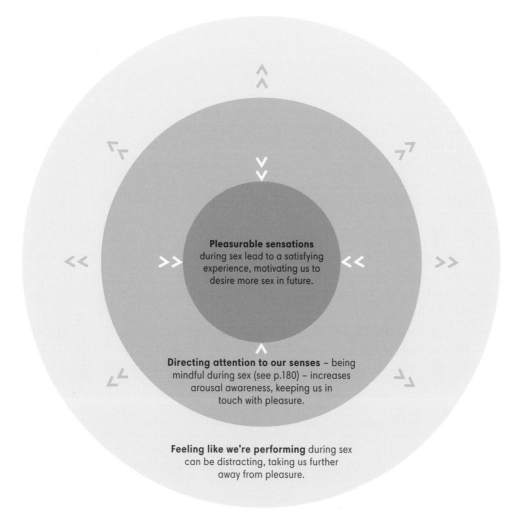

Pleasurable sensations during sex lead to a satisfying experience, motivating us to desire more sex in future.

Directing attention to our senses – being mindful during sex (see p.180) – increases arousal awareness, keeping us in touch with pleasure.

Feeling like we're performing during sex can be distracting, taking us further away from pleasure.

What's
mindful sex?

This involves consciously bringing your attention to your sexual experience without judgment or self-criticism, whether with yourself or a partner.

Mindful practice is about composure, bringing our attention to thoughts without bias or labelling them good or bad. This stops us fielding attention to intrusive thoughts that pull us into stress responses. Mindfulness exercises around sex may be especially beneficial where there are added barriers, for example, if desire is low or, for some, if painful sex distracts from pleasure.

Benefits for sex

Psychologist Dr Lori Brotto carried out research into the benefits of mindful sex for cancer patients. She discovered that when we focus our attention on physical sensations, not only can we increase our perception of our physical arousal, but also the level of arousal itself increases. Regular mindful practice activates the brain's attention centre and

BRINGING MINDFULNESS INTO YOUR LIFE AND SEXUAL PLEASURE

You can incorporate elements of mindfulness into your sex life even if you don't have an existing meditation or mindfulness practice. Bear in mind that mindfulness isn't a quick fix; making the following practices part of a daily routine can help you integrate mindfulness into your sexual experiences.

Notice everyday pleasures. Keep a pleasure journal. Note simple things that provide pleasure, whether it's a first sip of coffee, getting into a comfy bed, the sun on your face, the feel of a soft jumper, or a friend's hug. Noticing pleasure outside of sex helps us to be more aware of it during sex. Take a deep breath in each pleasurable moment to help you focus fully on the experience.

Allow instead of question. When you notice intrusive or interrupting thoughts, allow them to be there. A simple acknowledgment, saying to yourself, "It's a thought, not a fact" reminds you that you play a role in shaping your reality. We have thousands of thoughts daily; awareness of this helps us realize that we can't practically give each one our attention.

As we switch our attention away from distractions and towards sensations, we give ourselves more opportunity to boost desire and arousal.

quietens thoughts. A meta-analysis of 47 studies found that mindfulness programmes reduced the negative components of psychological stress, reducing levels of the stress hormone cortisol. Changes to our mood also play a critical role in our perception of stress, promoting desire and supporting our biological arousal response as we feel calmer and more present.

TANTRIC SEX

Tantra is an ancient philosophy that replaces being goal-oriented with spiritual, sensual, and intimate awareness. Tantric sex involves connection via breath, mindfulness, and eye contact, creating sensual intimacy.

Focus on your breath. Bringing attention to your breath helps you focus on what's happening in your body in the moment. Slow, deep breaths in and out send a signal to your parasympathetic nervous system to calm the body. Honing the ability to focus on your breath outside of sex can help you practice this during sex, so you can focus on the sensations you're experiencing.

Take your time. Much of our lives are goal-orientated, but this is counterintuitive with sex. Taking time with everyday tasks develops a mindset that during sex gives the body and mind a chance to build anticipation, desire, and arousal.

Engage your senses. Check in sensually daily with what you feel, smell, taste, hear, and see. This develops a tool to focus on the here and now.

Create your context for sex. Think about your environment to move focus away from the everyday and switch off. This might involve removing distracting objects; listening to music; putting your phone aside – or in another room; having a hot shower or bath; and making your to-do list for the next day so your mind can switch off.

Is **scheduling** sex **unsexy?**

Our popular narrative is that the best sex is spontaneous and that planned intimacy isn't as exciting. However, putting time in the diary to be together definitely doesn't have to be unsexy.

For many, finding the time for sex is a practicality as we fit it in around our everyday routines. This means that, whether partnered or solo, sex often happens when we get into bed at night. We may find we design a routine for sex around this, building in flexibility for days that don't go to plan. This informal scheduling can work well as, relaxed and wound down after the day, we're less likely to be distracted mentally and, as a result, more able to lean into responsive desire (see p.130), enjoying the opportunity for physical closeness.

A time for intimacy

It's important, though, not to schedule in sex as some type of goal. While anticipating sex can sometimes act as an aphrodisiac, feeding desire, if we're struggling with sex, scheduling it can create expectation and pressure, building anxiety and leading to avoidance.

It can also devalue other moments of intimacy, often non-sexual, which are valuable to relationships. Instead, think about putting aside time for physical closeness and connection, which may or may not lead to sex. Creating a habit to be together in this way is positive, as research shows that couples who consistently nurture physical intimacy report the highest levels of sexual satisfaction. The key is that they actively prioritize this time rather than expect it to just happen.

Sometimes, getting used to something, known as habituation (see p.63), can dampen erotic desire. If routine kills desire, small changes – to lighting, positions, location, or using lube or a sex toy – can be a psychological and physiological boost, rewarding us with a release of motivating dopamine (see p.56) to fuel desire as we break away from predictability.

So, is spontaneous sex better?

Often treated as the holy grail, spontaneous sex – or spontaneous desire (see p.130) – is most common when we first meet someone. The narrative is we're so turned on we can't contain ourselves and sex is passionate and hot. The counter-narrative is that the sex we have with a person over time is boring.

When we think about spontaneous sex in another way, it reflects how in the early stages of getting to know someone, typically there are higher levels of sexual currency (see p.220) – the attention we give each other outside of sex, such as kissing, eye contact, touch, and attention – which acts as a trigger for desire. Also, as routines aren't established in this "honeymoon phase", we use sex to build a connection. It's natural for sex to become more routine, but this doesn't mean it's less satisfying.

Whether sex is planned or unplanned, it's our focus on pleasure that counts.

Is **experience** important?

We've been socialized to place meaning on the number of sexual partners someone has had. However, this is a reductive way to evaluate sex.

Our conditioning tells us that how many sexual partners someone has had correlates with how sexually experienced and skilled they are.

We've also been socialized to place meaning on numbers of sexual partners, with assumptions around what's not enough, just right, or too much. As a result, we may have a negative self-perception if we think we've had too few or too many partners, as embedded messages tell us that this is in some way problematic.

A false barometer

The reality is that judging experience based on these popular narratives doesn't tell us anything about a person's sex life apart from the number of people they've had sexual experiences with. It doesn't tell us, for

A RECIPE FOR SATISFACTION
Good sex and confidence doesn't come from how many people we've slept with, but is about our approach to sex, being informed, and how we communicate.

Good communication with partners helps us to express our desires and listen to their needs.

Being well informed from trusted sources and healthy messaging gives us the confidence to talk to partners about sex.

Sexual satisfaction is a subjective measure and something that can ebb and flow throughout life.

Sex is a subjective experience, which we keep trying to measure objectively.

example, about the quality of the sex that either or all partners experienced, how satisfied they felt, or how long they've been sexually active for.

Sex is subjective, so trying to measure sexual "skill" in this way brings into question what counts as experience. Is it the number of times we've had intercourse? How many orgasms we've had? How many partners we've had – what if we've been with a partner for years? Also, if we're in a sexual relationship but not having intercourse, doesn't this count? Does solo sex count?

Constantly evolving

All sex is subjective, co-created in the moment – whether with different partners, the same partner in a different context, or on our own – and there's no single measure of what counts as experience. Knowing ourselves sexually and recognizing that sex evolves in a never-ending process of learning and developing (see p.218) is one of the best ways to feel sexually confident.

The removal of pressure to perform reduces concerns about lack of experience.

We feel increased confidence rather than fearing failure.

Not being goal-oriented allows us to focus on what we're feeling rather than a concept of success.

Is **Sexuality** *fluid?*

Sexuality has often been viewed as something that's fixed over a lifetime. Growing recognition of how sexuality can evolve is closing this gap in our understanding.

As we learn more about sexuality, we become aware of how heteronormative and mononormative – believing the "norm" is a relationship between two monogamous partners – our culture is. Over the past few decades, sexologists have challenged this thinking and helped us understand how sexuality can be far more nuanced than the binary definitions often given. In 1948, US sexologist Alfred Kinsey produced the "Kinsey Scale", published in *Sexual Behavior in the Human Male;* based on interviews with thousands of people, it explored people's sexual orientations. While it's considered limited today, this groundbreaking research set the path to challenging ideas that sexuality is binary and fixed. The Kinsey scale used a sliding scale labelled from "strictly heterosexual" to "strictly

homosexual", with varying levels of attraction to different sexes in between. Kinsey's research showed that sexual behaviours, thoughts, and feelings could be fluid; preferences weren't always fixed, and strict categorizations for sexual orientation were limiting.

Sexual orientation is a part of our identity and relates to our romantic and/or sexual attraction to others (see p.19). Today we understand increasingly there's a huge

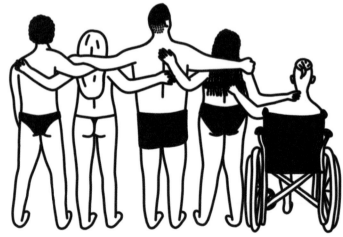

diversity of sexualities and that how someone describes their sexuality should be respected as their own identity.

Avoiding assumptions

We often draw conclusions about others' sexuality based on what we observe and without considering context. So, for example, if someone we thought was straight then has a same-sex partner, we may assume their sexuality has changed. What may not be apparent is that they identified as bisexual, but didn't feel comfortable expressing this before meeting the right person. Context is also critical where there are cultural and legal limitations on sexuality and its expression.

Another incorrect assumption is that when someone transitions or their gender identity changes, their sexual orientation has to change, too, for example, from heterosexual to gay. In reality, they may always have identified with one gender and their sexuality has stayed constant. Or their sexuality might be realized as fluid.

Understanding that erotic exploration – the areas we may explore in fantasies and pornography – is a separate concept from sexuality can also help us avoid assumptions about ourselves. For example, many who identify as straight watch same-sex pornography or have same-sex fantasies, but they may or may not feel a desire to act on these explorations in person.

Sexuality is nuanced and individual; for some, it can be fluid over the course of their life.

Do sexual comfort zones hold us back?

The gaps in our sexual lives represent the space between our reality and ideal. When we examine these gaps, we can find the motivation to make changes and enjoy increased satisfaction.

When we're stuck in an unhelpful pattern of sexual behaviour, such as faking pleasure or repeatedly having sex the same way, we're sticking within our familiar comfort zones. Understanding the psychology behind comfort zones can help us break out of these limiting patterns.

When we repeat unchallenging behaviour, our brains settle into the comfort of routine. Changing patterns means venturing into the unknown, signalling potential fear – and its associated psychological risks – to our brains. In this way, we can carry on having the same thoughts, feelings, and actions – reinforcing negative emotions, such as shame, anxiety, and self-consciousness.

A desire to change

To change behaviours that hold us back, we require motivation. Asking ourselves why we think we should change is the first step in becoming aware of potential barriers. We can then challenge automatic negative thoughts, which are often based on ingrained scripts and ideas, replacing these with positive alternatives. In this way, we can change our thinking around sex and motivate ourselves to broaden our perspectives.

New sexual horizons

When we find ways to close the gaps in our sexual lives – for example, by improving communication with partners, or recognizing social and cultural messages and distractions that can stop us enjoying sex fully – the more positive and accepting of our sexual selves we can be, and the more we can break away from feelings of shame (see p.32). In turn, we feel more confident being our authentic sexual selves and motivated to explore if we wish.

Exploring sexual comfort zones

Breaking away from comfort zones can take time. A practical exercise is to map out where you'd place certain sexual acts in a series of zones, graded "most comfortable" to "not at all comfortable". This can help you to think about where you might feel happiest starting to move out of a comfort zone, as well as areas that may not interest you at all.

COMFORT-ZONE QUESTIONS

What do I want?

What's getting in my way and how can I think about that differently?

When I try something new, how do I feel?

What have I learnt and can I continue to explore?

In the comfort zone, our brain settles into familiar patterns. We feel in control and safe, but sexually this might not equate to satisfaction and fulfilment.

In the fear zone, we can feel anxiety about changing a familiar behaviour, triggering the release of the stress hormone cortisol. We may doubt ourselves and worry about change.

In the learning zone, we can feel a sense of achievement over trying something new. As a result, the brain rewards us with a burst of dopamine (see p.56), fuelling motivation.

In the growth zone, self-limiting narratives are weakened and confidence grows. Encouraged, we explore more and are rewarded with dopamine again.

Sexual health

Our sexual health – physical and mental – is about far more than an absence of problems or infection. A key marker of good sexual health and wellbeing is how able we are to exercise informed choice in our sex lives. Being aware of our contraceptive choices and how to protect ourselves against sexually transmitted infections and unwanted pregnancy, as well as having sexual health checkups, puts us in control. In addition, understanding the relationship between our mental and sexual health – for some, complicated by past trauma – can help us navigate problems, make adaptations if needed, and regain sexual confidence.

What is sexual health?

The World Health Organization (WHO) defines sexual health as not just the absence of dysfunction or disease, but feeling "physical, emotional, mental, and social wellbeing" in relation to sex.

The WHO goes on to describe the importance of a positive and respectful approach to sex and the ability to enjoy safe and pleasurable relationships without "coercion, discrimination, and violence". This sexual health definition takes a holistic approach, encompassing our physical, mental, and social contexts.

Informed choices

One of the key elements of this definition is choice. A huge part of our sexual wellbeing is about being able to make informed sexual choices about what we want our sex lives and relationships to look like. This is a two-step process involving first, gaining trustworthy information, then choosing what to do with it. Once well-informed, this helps us consider sex from a less judgmental and more inclusive position.

Information is of course context- and culture-dependent, often shaped by religion and faith. The proliferation of the internet has made sexual information widely and easily accessible, and many turn to online sources to educate themselves. Often, though, information gleaned online is inaccurate and/or misleading. Being well-informed therefore means gathering and seeking out information from trustworthy sources. These can help you understand what sex can involve and how it works; how sexually transmitted infections (STIs) are spread; and what your contraceptive choices are. If you need support, find trusted people to talk to and try to be proactive about sexual-health checkups.

Being well-informed can help you communicate with partners so you're better able to express your desires and preferences. You can work out what you need to feel safe and comfortable sexually, and may be prompted to think about why you want a sexual experience and whether it's the right reason for you.

Comfortable situations

A key part of sexual health is being happy with the situation you're in. Sex should always happen with your free will and without any

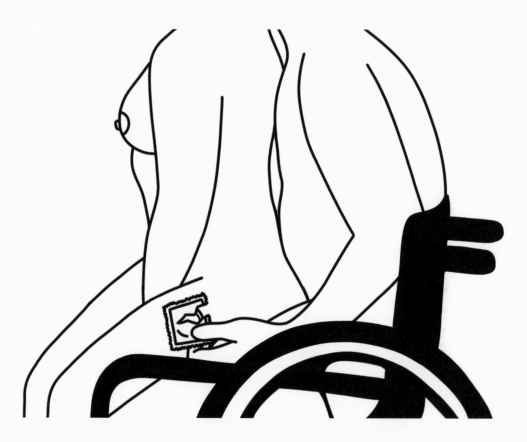

type of coercion (see p.20); it shouldn't take place under pressure – whether from a partner or peers – for example, to have sex without protection or because you feel you *should* to fit in with everyone else. You should always feel you can change your mind, and happy that you've been able to consider protection in advance of sex.

Positive reasons for having sex include mutual attraction; desire; a wish for intimacy and/or pleasure; and curiosity. Always ensure it's your personal decision and that you're aware of potential consequences.

Sex should always be legal, consensual, and without coercion.

Has our definition of virginity moved on?

As our ideas about sex have evolved, this has left traditional concepts about what virginity is lodged in the past. Today, virginity can mean different things to different people.

The widely accepted definition of virginity still focuses on first-time intercourse. However, this definition only covers one part of sex and excludes the experiences of many, such as those having non-heterosexual experiences, or whose preferences or ability don't involve intercourse. This traditional view of what virginity is also leans into the model of goal-orientated, linear sex (see p.13), failing to encompass ideas about sexual exploration.

The concept of virginity

The sense of expectation many of us have about "losing our virginity" often revolves around the thought that the later you leave it after the age of consent, and the less in line with your peers, the less "normal" you are.

What's key is that we understand that the concept of sexual experience is subjective and person-dependent. The most important thing for our sexual debuts, whatever they look like for us, is that they're at a time of our choosing and are legal, consensual, and safe.

Our definition of virginity is narrowly focused around intercourse.

How likely is pregnancy after sex?

Correctly used, contraceptive methods have high protection rates (see p.200), but if you have regular unprotected sex, pregnancy is a consideration.

WHAT ABOUT HYMENS?

There is a lot of misinformation about the hymen – a thin piece of tissue at the vaginal opening. One common misconception is that the hymen only breaks when people with vaginas first have sex. In reality, it can change, break, or wear away over time, from activities such as using tampons, exercise, and masturbating. Many aren't aware or don't notice when it breaks; some who may experience light bleeding often assume it's period-related.

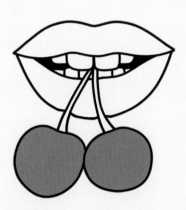

Each person's fertility depends on multiple factors, including age, lifestyle, and frequency of intercourse. After ejaculation into the vagina, sperm can live in the reproductive tract for up to five days, so during that time there's the potential for fertilization if a sperm reaches an egg.

The timing of intercourse impacts the chance of getting pregnant. The days leading up to ovulation, and up to 24 hours after ovulation – which on average occurs around day 14 of a cycle – are most fertile, as once an egg is released, it moves down the fallopian tube where it can be fertilized by sperm. There's very little chance of getting pregnant outside of this fertile window; however, as cycle lengths can vary widely, and for some are irregular, estimating this is not a reliable method of contraception on its own.

The most common way for people to get pregnant is through intercourse, but there's a chance of pregnancy if sperm comes into contact with the vagina, for example, if your partner ejaculates close to the vaginal opening.

Is talking about protection a **passion killer?**

No – safe sex is great sex. The assumption that a conversation about protection will dampen desire is likely to be based on our awkwardness in talking openly and honestly about sex.

An important part of sex is feeling safe in the knowledge – not the assumption – that you aren't taking risks with your health. We often hear phrases such as, "They don't seem like the type to have an STI" or, "I trust them" or, "They said it's fine", but these are emotive rather than factual statements.

Avoiding assumptions

Feeling that you can trust someone isn't a safe way to decide their sexual health status. Nor does someone's sexual history necessarily indicate their likelihood of being infected with an STI (see p.204). In addition, some STIs are asymptomatic, so however healthy someone seems, this isn't an indicator of whether they're currently STI-free. The reality is that anyone having unprotected sex is at risk of contracting an STI from partners.

Thinking about contraception

Discussing contraception is about considering the best choices for your body. If you're thinking about taking hormonal contraception, finding the method that works for you and your health is key. If a contraceptive method doesn't protect against STIs, you may need to discuss using condoms with a partner until you've both had a sexual health screening. If you're sexually exclusive with a partner, you can then choose when to stop using condoms.

Celebrating sexual health

Looking after our sexual health is like looking after any other aspect of our wellbeing, and is something to be celebrated rather than ashamed of. Talking about protection, and giving consent on the basis of agreed protection (see p.21), is about ensuring safety

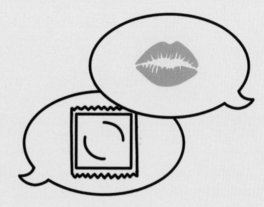

during sex. This should be seen by all as showing care and responsibility for everyone's health. This sense of personal responsibility and the confidence to discuss it can be a good sign for other elements of a relationship. It opens up a space for honest communication when it comes to sex, which in itself can benefit our sex lives (see p.20).

Talking to a new partner about protection before getting into a sexual situation, rather than having the discussion just before sex, can be ideal. This helps you assess how much importance they place on the topic and if they accept your personal boundaries.

Feeling confident in your own and your partner's sexual health can help you relax and, ultimately, have better sex. Feeling safe can mean you're less inhibited and more able to focus on pleasurable sensations, rather than being distracted by sexual health worries.

STARTING THE CONVERSATION

The following suggestions may be helpful if you feel awkward asking about protection.

"Before things go further, I just wanted to let you know I'm on the pill, but until we've both had a sexual health screening I'd feel more comfortable using condoms, too. Once the results come back shall we discuss it again?"

"I like to test between each partner as a way to keep us both safe. Would you be happy to do the same?"

"I haven't found the right hormonal contraception for me yet, so in the meantime, please can we use condoms?"

"I don't want us to risk a pregnancy now, so using contraception feels really important. What are your thoughts?"

What are the options for safe sex?

Using protection during sex offers us choice and autonomy over our sex lives. Knowing what's available and how each type of protection works will help you choose what's best for you.

Natural or artificial methods of protection prevent STI transmission and/or pregnancy. STIs and unintended pregnancy are the main negative consequences of unprotected sex; psychologically, being unprotected can also cause anxiety. The main types of protection, outlined below and detailed on pages 200–201, comprise barrier methods and hormonal and non-hormonal contraception. Other options include surgery and emergency contraception. For trans people, protection depends on individual circumstances, so consult a medical professional for personalized advice.

TYPES OF PROTECTION

Barrier methods
These mainly comprise condoms, the cap, and the diaphragm. Condoms create a physical barrier, preventing sperm entering the vagina and subsequently fertilizing an egg. Condoms also protect against STIs, as do dental dams, which are worn over the vulva or anus during oral sex. The cap and the diaphragm protect against pregnancy, but not STIs.

Hormonal contraception
These include the pill; injections, implants, or patches; the vaginal ring; and hormonal coil. They involve taking synthetic hormones to stop ovulation, thin the womb lining, and thicken cervical mucus. The combined pill and vaginal ring contain oestrogen and aren't advised with some medications and for those aged over 35 who also smoke, where cardiovascular and other health risks are increased.

Intrauterine methods (IUS and IUD)
Popularly referred to as "the coil", these are implanted into the uterus to make it a harder environment for sperm to fertilize an egg. There are hormonal and non-hormonal options. IUDs and IUSs don't protect against STIs, so barrier methods may be needed.

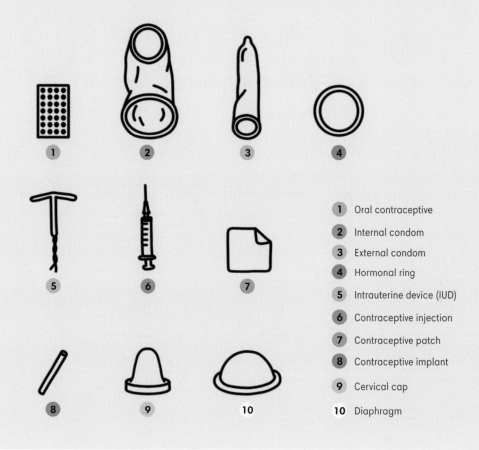

1 Oral contraceptive

2 Internal condom

3 External condom

4 Hormonal ring

5 Intrauterine device (IUD)

6 Contraceptive injection

7 Contraceptive patch

8 Contraceptive implant

9 Cervical cap

10 Diaphragm

Natural family planning

Also called fertility awareness, this involves tracking signs of ovulation – the most fertile time in the menstrual cycle – and planning intercourse around these days to either prevent or get pregnant. This may be preferred for religious reasons or to avoid hormonal methods of contraception.

Surgical contraception

Also referred to as sterilization, these are permanent surgical changes to the body to prevent pregnancy. A vasectomy cuts or seals the vas deferens (the tubes that carry sperm from the testicles to the penis, see pp.100–101) to stop sperm getting into semen. Tubal ligation is the procedure to block or seal the fallopian tubes to prevent sperm reaching and fertilizing an egg.

Emergency contraception

Often used as a result of failed contraception, such as a condom breaking, this can be either a pill taken after sex or the fitting of an IUD. The "morning-after pill" can be taken up to five days after sex; the sooner it's taken, the more effective it is. Or an IUD can be fitted by a medical professional up to five days after sex to prevent pregnancy; it can then stay in as ongoing contraception.

Which protection is best for me?

BARRIER METHODS	HOW TO USE
The cap and the diaphragm are circular domes made of soft, thin silicone. They act as a barrier to the cervix so sperm can't reach the uterus.	Used with spermicide (to kill sperm), it is inserted into the vagina before sex and left in for at least six hours after sex. A health practitioner will show you how to insert one.
Condoms are made from very thin latex, polyurethane, or polyisoprene (see p.202).	External condoms are worn over the penis during vaginal, anal, or oral sex. Internal condoms are worn inside the vagina, placed before contact with a penis.

HORMONAL CONTRACEPTION

The combined pill, or "the pill", contains oestrogen and progestogen.	There are several versions of the pill, but it's usually taken once a day for 21 days with a seven day break, during which time there's a period-like bleed.
The progestogen-only pill, also called the "mini pill", contains progestogen only.	This is taken daily without a break. Depending on the type, it needs to be taken within three or 12 hours of a set time. Periods may stop, be lighter, or more frequent or irregular.
The contraceptive implant is a small, plastic rod that releases progestogen into the bloodstream.	The implant is placed under the skin by a medical professional. A long-term hormonal contraception, it's useful for those who struggle to remember to take a daily pill.
The contraceptive injection releases progestogen into the bloodstream.	The injection is given by a medical professional. As with implants, this long-term hormonal contraception is useful for those who struggle to remember to take a daily pill.
The contraceptive patch is worn on the skin, delivering hormones transdermally, that is, via the skin.	A patch lasts one week. After three weeks, you have a week off, during which time there may be a period-like bleed.
The vaginal ring is a soft, plastic ring that releases a continuous dose of progestogen and oestrogen.	This is placed inside the vagina, usually for 21 days with a seven-day break, during which time there may be a period-like bleed. Can be worn during intercourse.
The intrauterine system (IUS), or hormonal coil, is a T-shaped plastic device that releases progestogen.	This is inserted into the uterus by a medical professional.

NON-HORMONAL CONTRACEPTION

The intrauterine device (IUD), or coil, is a T-shaped copper and plastic device that releases copper, which alters cervical mucus to make it hard for sperm to live.	This is inserted into the uterus by a medical professional.
Natural family planning is a self-monitored way to check fertility signs through the menstrual cycle to see when pregnancy is most likely.	Body temperature, changes to cervical mucus, and length of cycle are used to estimate ovulation. If used as contraception, sex is avoided around this time.

The method you choose depends on your needs – whether you wish to avoid pregnancy and/or need protection against STIs. With some hormonal contraceptives, factors such as age, health, and lifestyle are considered (see p.198).

HOW LONG IT LASTS	PROTECTION OFFERED	WILL IT WORK?
Typically, one year. After sex, it's washed in warm water and mild soap, dried, and left in a container until its next use.	Protects against pregnancy, but not against STIs, so condoms may be needed.	Used correctly with spermicide, it's 92–96 per cent effective at preventing pregnancy.
These are single-use. If switching from anal to vaginal or oral sex, use a new condom to avoid transferring bacteria.	Condoms are the only contraceptive method that protect against both pregnancy and STIs.	External condoms are 98 per cent effective at preventing pregnancy; internal condoms 95 per cent.
Provides contraception for as long as it's being taken.	Protects against pregnancy, but not STIs, so condoms may be needed.	Taken correctly, the combined pill is over 99 per cent effective in preventing pregnancy.
Provides contraception for as long as it's being taken.	Protects against pregnancy, but not STIs, so condoms may be needed.	Taken correctly, the mini pill is 99 per cent effective in preventing pregnancy.
Lasts for up to three years, but can be removed at any time if you wish.	Protects against pregnancy, but not STIs, so condoms may be needed.	Implants are 99 per cent effective in preventing pregnancy.
Lasts for 8–13 weeks.	Protects against pregnancy, but not STIs, so condoms may be needed.	Injections are 99 per cent effective in preventing pregnancy.
Provides contraception for as long as it's being used.	Protects against pregnancy, but not STIs, so condoms may be needed.	Used correctly, it's 99 per cent effective in preventing pregnancy.
Provides contraception for as long as it's being used.	Protects against pregnancy, but not STIs, so condoms may be needed.	Used correctly, it's 99 per cent effective in preventing pregnancy.
Lasts for 3–5 years, but can be removed at any point.	Protects against pregnancy, but not STIs, so condoms may be needed.	Inserted correctly, it's 99 per cent effective in preventing pregnancy.
Lasts for 5–10 years, but can be removed at any point.	Protects against pregnancy, but not STIs, so condoms may be needed.	Inserted correctly, it's 99 per cent effective in preventing pregnancy.
An on-going method.	Aims to protect against pregnancy, not STIs, so condoms may be needed.	Used consistently and accurately, it's 99 per cent effective. Advice from a fertility awareness teacher is advised.

Which **condom** should I choose?

The array of condoms available can make selecting one a confusing task. Knowing what different condoms offer can help you choose.

The most commonly used condoms are external ones worn over the penis, which come in a range of shapes, sizes, and materials.

- **Condoms are latex or non-latex.** All are lubricated to make them easy to put on the penis, but extra lube can be used for added pleasure or comfort. If you add lube to a latex condom, it needs to be water- or silicone-based, as oil-based lube can cause them to break (see p.86). Non-latex condoms are available for those with a latex allergy, made with either polyurethane – a synthetic plastic, or polyisoprene – a synthetic non-latex rubber. Non-latex condoms can be used with all lubricants.
- **Textured condoms** have raised ridges or dots for added sensation.
- **Ultra-thin condoms** are designed for extra sensitivity.
- **Flavoured condoms** are intended primarily for oral sex, to disguise the taste of latex. Bear in mind that some coatings contain glycerine, which can contribute to vaginal yeast infection if worn during intercourse.

HOW TO PUT ON A CONDOM

Condoms are stretchy, so standard-sized ones fit most penises. However, if they're too loose or too tight, this can make them less effective, so check for bigger or smaller sizes if needed. When you put on a condom:

- Take care not to tear it when removing it from the packet – it's best not to use your teeth!

- Place it over the tip of the erect penis, using thumb and forefinger to squeeze air out of the teat, then gently roll the condom down to the penis base.

- When removing, hold the condom at the base of the penis so it doesn't come off as the penis withdraws, which could cause contact with semen if this leaked out.

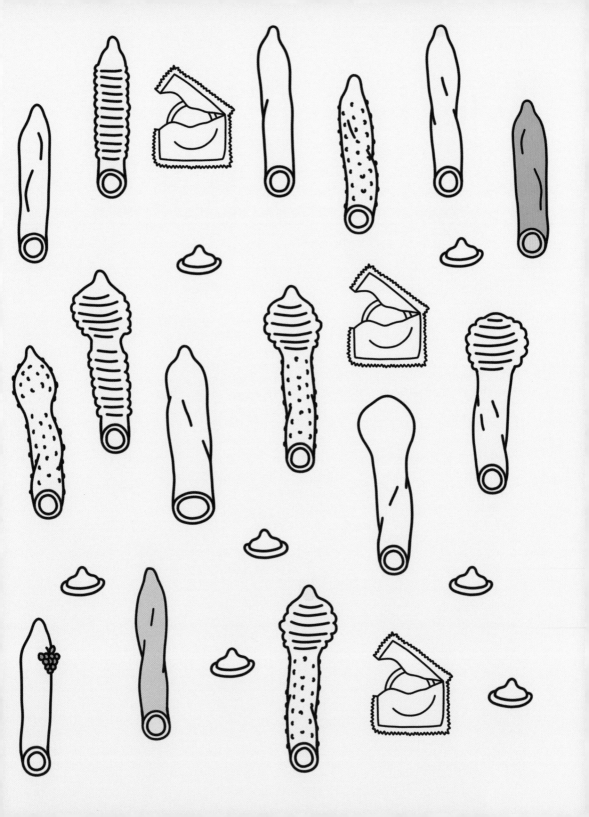

Will I know if I have an STI?

Sexually transmitted infections (STIs) may cause symptoms. However, it's important to know that all STIs can be present without causing any symptoms at all.

You can contract a bacterial, viral, or parasitic STI via vaginal, anal, or oral sex. Common STIs include human papillomavirus (HPV) (see opposite); chlamydia; gonorrhoea; syphilis; genital warts; genital herpes; trichomoniasis; pubic lice (crabs); scabies; and human immunodeficiency virus (HIV), which, if untreated, can lead to acquired immune deficiency syndrome (AIDS).

What are the symptoms?
Common symptoms include:

- **Pain** when urinating.
- **A change in vaginal discharge**, or an unusual discharge from the penis, vagina, or anus.
- **Unusual vaginal bleeding**.
- **Blisters, warts, or sores** around the genitals or anus.
- **A rash**.
- **Lumps or growths** around the anus or genitals.
- **Itching or discomfort** around the genitals or anus.

WORLDWIDE INFECTION RATES
In one year, the World Health Organisation estimated 374 million new infections of four common STIs:

Infection rates in 2020
- Chlamydia (129 million)
- Gonorrhoea (82 million)
- Syphilis (7.1 million)
- Trichomoniasis (156 million)

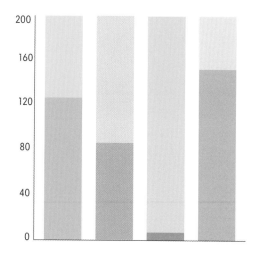

As all STIs may be asymptomatic, people may not realize they're infected. For example, chlamydia, a common bacterial infection, is often symptomless. It's easy to treat with a short course of antibiotics. However, if left untreated, it can spread, with potential long-term health consequences, particularly in those assigned female at birth (AFAB), where it can lead to pelvic inflammatory disease (PID), increased risk of ectopic pregnancy (a non-viable pregnancy where the egg implants in a fallopian tube), and infertility. It's never too late to test for chlamydia as potential further damage can be halted.

Some infections, such as genital warts and HIV, are incurable, but can be well managed with treatment and medication, so it's important to get tested.

Telling partners

If you test positive for an STI, you should inform all recent sexual partners (since your last sexual health screening) so they can get tested. Some clinics offer an anonymous "partner notification" service, where they'll inform partners without identifying you.

HUMAN PAPILLOMAVIRUS (HPV)

This is one of the most common STIs. In one year alone (2018), there were around 43 million infections in the US. There are more than 100 types of HPV. Usually, it's symptomless, but it can cause genital warts, and some high-risk HPV viruses are linked to abnormal cell changes that can develop into cancer – specifically cervical, penile, anal, oropharyngeal, vaginal, and vulva cancers.

Cervical screening programmes, which take a sample of cells from the cervix, help to detect cell changes that can lead to cervical cancer. If you test positive, the cells can be treated before becoming cancerous. In the UK, people with a cervix are invited for a screening from the age of 25 to 49, every three years; then from 50 to 64, every five years.

In 2006, an HPV vaccine was approved. In the UK, this is routinely offered to all children aged 12–13. A review of worldwide data on over 60 million young people showed an 83 per cent reduction in high-risk HPV in teenage girls and a 66 per cent reduction in women aged 20–24, indicating the programme's success.

When should I have a sexual health **check?**

If you're having unprotected sex, testing between each partner can avoid passing on a sexually transmitted infection (STI), so is a simple way to look after your own and a partner's health.

Sexual health checks help you take control of your health; minimize the risk of spreading infection; and give peace of mind. The rule of thumb is to get checked between partners; if you engage in high-risk activities and/or have sex with new partners without protection, testing every 3-6 months is advisable. There's also a range of other reasons for screening.

- If a partner or previous partner says they have an STI.
- If you're in a relationship and want to move from condoms to a contraception that doesn't protect against STIs, best practice is for all parties to be checked.
- If you've had sex with someone and are unsure of their status.
- If you're trying to conceive. Some STIs can impact fertility. Infections can also cause potential complications during pregnancy that can affect the unborn baby.

Getting tested

Sexual health clinics, sometimes known as GUM (genitourinary medicine) clinics, specialize in sexual health testing, and GP surgeries test for STIs. Home-testing kits are also available,

but the gold standard is to be checked by a sexual health professional.

Without judgment, you'll be asked a series of questions about your lifestyle and medical and sexual history, alongside recent sexual encounters and if you're experiencing symptoms. You may have a blood test and will be asked for a sample, which may be a urine sample; or a vaginal, penis, or anal swab. In most cases, you can take these yourself in the toilet. You may also have a genital examination. The clinic will usually give you your results within a few days. If any result is positive, you'll be prescribed antibiotics or medication to manage the infection.

How quickly do infections show up?

There's a window of time between catching an infection and it showing up on a test. This means if you think you have an STI, you'll have to wait until this period has passed to be sure you're clear. For chlamydia and gonorrhoea, it's two weeks; for HIV, UK guidelines state it's 45 days for laboratory tests; 90 days for rapid tests. If you think you've been exposed to HIV, post-exposure prophylaxis medication (PEP) can reduce your risk (see opposite).

Managing HIV today

Since the HIV/AIDS crisis of the 1980s, there have been incredible developments in treatments. Today, anti-retroviral medications help control the viral load – the amount of virus in the blood – of someone with HIV, reducing levels to undetectable amounts. When HIV is undetectable, this means it's untransmittable (see below). For those without HIV who risk exposure, treatments known as pre-exposure prophylaxis (PrEP) and post-exposure prophylaxis (PEP) can offer protection against contracting HIV.

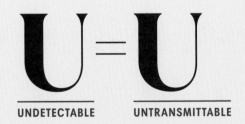

UNDETECTABLE **UNTRANSMITTABLE**

The U=U concept is an international campaign to raise awareness about the scientific data that proves people living with HIV who take effective anti-retroviral therapy cannot transmit the virus to sexual partners.

- **PEP** is a 28-day course of medication that must start to be taken within 72 hours (ideally within 24) after possible exposure to HIV. This is a combination of HIV drugs that can stop the infection taking hold. PEP is designed for emergency use rather than as a regular method of preventing transmission and it is not a cure for HIV.
- **PrEP** is taken in advance of sexual contact, where you might be at risk of contracting HIV. Unlike PEP, it's designed to be taken in a regular and planned way; research shows that when taken correctly, PrEP is highly efficient at preventing HIV transmission.

All of these treatments challenge many of the assumptions about passing on HIV. They mean that you're more likely to catch the virus from someone who doesn't know that they have it, rather than someone who is taking medication correctly to manage it, emphasizing the importance of testing and education.

When should I have a sexual health check? **207**

Does our
mental health
impact sex?

Our mental health and sexual wellbeing can be seen as having a bidirectional relationship – with the status of each often having a significant impact on the other.

There are many ways in which mental health problems, such as depression and anxiety, can influence our sex lives. For example, symptoms of depression such as fatigue, low mood, and shame can decrease sexual interest and motivation for sex (see opposite). Likewise, issues such as erectile dysfunction and painful sex (see pp.120–123), can contribute to poor mental health.

A source of distraction
Problems such as chronic fatigue and anxiety can affect our ability to stay focused on pleasure and arousal; when our brain is diverted from pleasure, this impacts the physiological arousal process (see pp.92–93) and the body's ability to respond physically, potentially causing problems such as lack of lubrication or erection issues. When sex doesn't go to plan, this can have a cyclical effect, feeding into feelings of negativity and shame. Talking to a partner if possible about how these feelings affect you can avoid assumptions and allow you to work together to overcome issues.

Looking at medication
The group of antidepressants known as selective serotonin reuptake inhibitors (SSRIs), often used to treat depression, can themselves cause challenges with sexual desire and functioning (see opposite). This means it can be difficult to work out whether sexual dysfunction is caused by the depression or the medication, or is a combination of the two.

However, the improvements to mental health that medication can bring are associated with increased overall wellbeing, which has a positive impact on our sex lives. When health practitioners clearly explain potential side effects, it's possible to navigate any changes. Instead of seeing side effects as a complete roadblock to your sex life, making adaptations, such as leaning into practices that build pleasure and sensation, can make sex work for you.

Our mental health status can have a range of knock-on effects on our sex lives.

Low mood, lack of confidence, and low self-esteem can lead to negative and intrusive thoughts, which can be huge interrupters of sexual arousal and desire.

Feelings of shame may arise if you feel unable to disclose or discuss with your partner how you're feeling. This can increase feelings of isolation, or worries about what they're thinking.

Fatigue, a common symptom of depression, can leave you feeling drained and tired cognitively, emotionally, and physically, which can push sex to the bottom of the priority list.

SSRI medications for depression (see opposite) increase serotonin levels in the brain, which can interfere with sexual function. A commonly reported side effect is a dampening impact on sexual arousal, leading to problems such as delayed ejaculation and delayed or absent orgasm.

How can
sexual trauma
impact sex?

Trauma can have a profound impact on someone's sex life, mental health, and physical wellbeing. Finding resources to help you cope can be key for regaining sexual confidence.

Trauma that can affect our sex lives can come in many forms, from assault, abuse, and violence, to experiences such as traumatic surgery, injury, or birth trauma. It can also include emotional trauma, for example, after a betrayal.

Experiencing trauma leads to significant psychological wounds. It's very possible for these wounds to heal, though reaching a place of greater peace after trauma takes time. There's no standardized response, so it's important to focus on your own healing process.

Trauma and our brains

Research reveals that traumatic events have wide-ranging impacts on brain function. As well as affecting areas connected to memory, such as the hippocampus, amygdala, and prefrontal cortex, studies show that trauma can impact the brain's neurochemical system, leading to higher levels of the stress hormones noradrenaline and cortisol.

Where trauma leads to post-traumatic stress disorder (PTSD), studies show that levels of stress hormones can remain high over time. This helps explain why some who've experienced trauma describe feeling prolonged emotional reactivity with hypervigilant responses (see opposite).

Feeling in control

Each person's experience is subjective and context-dependent, and our responses are impacted by our psychological makeup, as well as previous life experience. However, a common feeling associated with trauma is of a sense of being out of control. Physical, emotional, and social responses are driven by a need to protect ourselves and regain control. Integrating healthy coping skills into your life (see pp.212–213) can help you learn how to manage.

Experiencing trauma can increase sensitivity to our unique triggers that remind us of the trauma. Repeated exposure to triggers can decrease our emotional tolerance to them. The brain reacts defensively, responding as if under threat.

We can become hyper-vigilant and hyper-sensitive. For example, sexualized or unpredictable touch, or touch initiated by someone else, can feel associated with past trauma, even if it's not a threat in the moment.

OUR TRAUMA RESPONSE

Being aware of how trauma might affect our responses can help us think about the steps we can take to interrupt negative cycles, and build strategies to help us navigate triggers and enjoy our sexual lives.

A state of hyper-arousal can lead to conditions such as post-traumatic stress disorder (PTSD), prolonging the stressed state, increasing alertness, and leading to flashbacks.

We may avoid certain situations or actions, such as opportunities for touch. This can affect relationships and create a negative cycle of behaviour and responses that exacerbate the original trauma.

How do I work through sexual trauma?

Regaining a sense of control after sexual trauma is about self-compassion and communication. It's important to take the time needed to rebuild trust and feel comfortable with intimacy.

Support from a trained professional if this is an option, and/or trusted friends, family, and support groups can be helpful. Exploring self-help strategies and working on communicating with a partner can also help you regain sexual trust.

Regaining control

Rebuilding a positive relationship with your body and how it interacts with sex can help you feel in control during sex. Self-guided touch combined with grounding techniques such as deep breathing can help re-familiarize you with your body. This might involve trying types and styles of touch to navigate what and where feels okay. When you feel ready, you can invite a partner to try this with you (see opposite).

Generally, strategies such as focused breathing can help you adjust to increased sensitivity after trauma. Other simple, accessible steps to help you navigate triggers and feel in control may include watching your drink being made, keeping a light on, or carrying a grounding sensory object.

Communicating with partners

A hyper-vigilant state after sexual trauma (see pp.210–211) can mean we have strong reactions to triggers that can impact our ability to be sexual or sensual with someone. We may lean into avoidance behaviours, such as evading touch, to manage challenging emotions. Communication is crucial. Being clear with a partner is the only way they can understand fully what's happening, and being able to express the need to stop or change something is important for you to feel in control of an experience. Unambiguous boundaries – which may have altered after trauma – not only help you both cope in the moment, they also allow you to rebuild trust so you can manage and enjoy consensual non-threatening experiences.

It can be challenging and scary to open up to a partner about past trauma. However, not explaining what happened risks you being re-traumatized if they fail to understand your boundaries and/or give you the time you need. This can have a knock-on impact on the wellbeing of you and your partner. Thinking ahead about how you'll approach this conversation can be helpful.

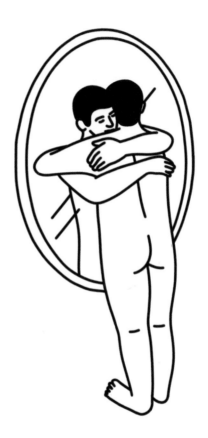

- Try focusing on how you are currently and how you experience the impact of past trauma in the here and now.
- Don't feel you need to go into detail or feel pressured to do so if you don't wish to. Disclose what feels appropriate.
- Try to focus on the specifics of what you can both do when you feel triggered or have a flashback.
- Be clear about any areas you don't want touched, or if there's anything you really want to avoid. Your partner isn't a mind-reader – even if something feels obvious to you, communicate it explicitly.
- Take time to build trust and intimacy – recognizing you'll have good days and bad days. You may wish to build up to a full sexual relationship, finding ways to connect and be intimate that work for you. A practical exercise is to place your hand over a partner's and guide them to where feels comfortable so they understand your

boundaries. If touch is triggering, advice and guidance from a professional therapist may be needed first to help you manage emotions and responses as they arise. The more you associate feelings with safety, pleasure, and connection, the safer you'll feel exploring and being sexual again.

Am I thinking about sex
too much?

How often we think about sex varies from person to person, but having sexual thoughts is very normal. However, if they start to feel intrusive, you may feel you need strategies to manage them.

It's not uncommon for sex to come into our consciousness at times when we're not having sex or purposefully thinking about it. We may be triggered by something in our environment that our brain has coded as sexually relevant; or we may think about sex, or even notice arousal, after associating a physical experience with pleasure – for example, the vibrations of a car, or sensation of water on our genitals in the shower.

Usually, thinking about sex a lot isn't a worry, but if thoughts are connected to concerns about sex, or they feel linked to strong impulses, this can become problematic.

Worries and preoccupations

Many of us have worries about sex, which may be to do with our bodies, the act of sex, or a partner's perception of us. If these become a preoccupation, anxiety and stress can impact our sex lives.

Our anxiety can be exacerbated by the fact that we live in a culture where it isn't easy to express our sexual concerns. This means that often when we experience worries, we don't know who to turn to and can feel isolated, which in turn adds to embarrassment and feelings of shame.

When thoughts become intrusive

If thoughts about sexual sensations or activities start to feel intrusive, obsessive, or that they can't be controlled, this can impact our mental wellbeing and relationships. We can avoid situations that we think act as triggers, and shame and self-criticism can cause feelings of distress that can interrupt our intimate relationships.

Some find they think obsessively about the contamination risk and/or risk of infection from the exchange of bodily fluids, which can affect their ability to be sexual with another person.

If sexual thoughts feel out of control or compulsive, it may be helpful to seek support and advice from a medical professional and/or qualified psychosexual therapist. They can help you identify triggers and find strategies to ground your thoughts away from sex when this isn't relevant, helping to release you from stuck patterns of thinking.

Trying not to think about sex can have the opposite effect, bringing it into our consciousness more.

How
sex
evolves

Throughout our lives, our definition of sex is constantly reshaped and adapted as our context shifts. We may be entering a new life phase – perhaps starting a family, experiencing natural ageing processes, or moving on after a breakup; or our relationships may be affected by infidelity, distance, or simply changing dynamics. As the meaning of sex in our lives evolves, embracing changes and being open to the concept of life-long sexual learning can help us to continue moving forwards, keeping sex relevant in our lives.

How do we stay sexually **curious?**

Our relationship with sex constantly evolves. Curiosity can be a key part of this process, allowing us to be open to new thoughts, feelings, and practices if we desire.

Curiosity is a critical component of our sex lives and one of the best tools we have for sparking desire. When curious, we're open to discovery; conversely, when we feel we know all we need to, we may think we can set aside curiosity, which can stifle desire.

Flexing our curiosity can strengthen sexual relationships and expand our perspective. In anticipation of trying something new, our brain rewards us with a motivating dopamine hit (see p.56), making us feel good and nudging us to continue exploring.

Lifelong learning

Our sexual learning never ends. As our life changes, so might our interests, influenced by our environment, situations, and contexts. There may of course be times when we don't feel sexually curious; but at points in our lives, we may feel ready for something that we didn't previously. Nurturing a sense of curiosity can mean we're receptive to trying something new. This doesn't have to mean going wildly out of your sexual comfort zone – unless you desire that; it may simply mean being open to the possibility of learning something different about yourself or your partner.

Working with change

When our lives shift – environmentally, psychologically, emotionally, and biologically – we adapt and develop. For some, how we experience sex can change during our lives. For example, if we go through trauma, pain, or injury, whether physical or psychological, we may need to adapt our sex lives so they work in our new situation. When we change partners we also adapt as we experience each partner slightly differently. Our sexual orientation can be fluid, too, rather than fixed throughout our lives (see p.186). Harnessing our curiosity can be an important force in our ever-changing sex lives.

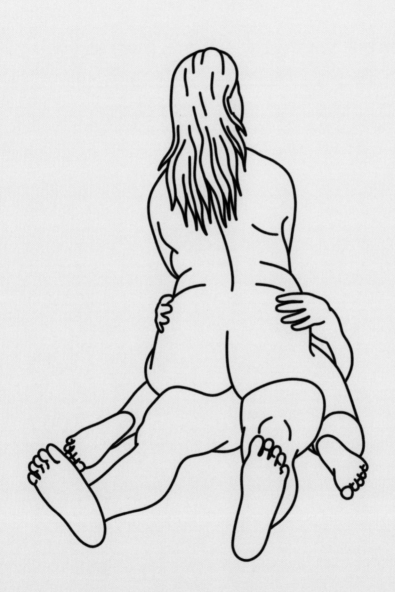

How do we keep a
connection going?

When couples feel disconnected, it can often be because they only engage affectionately as a precursor to sex, rather than maintaining sexual connection at other times.

Sexual currency – the sexual communication tool we use to connect with partners outside of sexual experiences, for example, with extended hugs, lingering kisses, flirting, eye contact, affirming compliments, playful touch, and suggestive messages – is different to physical affection. It's also one of the things commonly described as missing by couples who are struggling with their sexual connection.

A bridge between desire and sex

Sexual currency is about offering reminders of attraction and desire. If we think of it like a muscle, we need to flex it regularly to keep it toned and maintained – even if we aren't doing regular workouts. When we keep our sexual currency in credit, this fuels desire. We can also think of these acts of affection as the bridge between each sexual experience, maintaining a level of closeness between partners, rather than leaving a distance that can be harder to negotiate desire across.

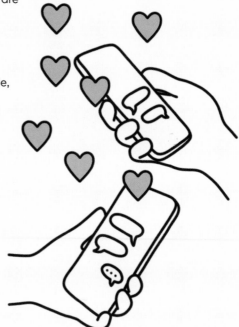

When currency runs low

Sexual currency tends to fluctuate between partners. Initially, it's often high, hand in hand with spontaneous desire. There may be constant reassurances and demonstrations of desire.

When couples feel sexually stuck, it's often because they show affection only as a prelude to sex and fail to maintain a connection at other times. Once we're aware of this we can deliberately change our behaviour. Anecdotally, couples who work on and improve sexual currency report a positive impact on their sex lives.

Emotional communication

An extension of sexual currency is the concept of "bids for attention". Relationship therapist Dr John Gottman developed this concept when he analyzed couple's interactions, then met with them six years later to see who was together, who'd broken up, or who was together but seemingly not happy. He described bids for attention as a "fundamental unit of emotional communication". Bids are verbal or non-verbal, big or small, and signal a need for attention. Examples include asking how a partner's day went or enjoying a quick hug, to helping with a problem when asked. When a partner makes a bid for attention we

can either acknowledge it and turn towards them, for example, by stopping what we're doing and answering a question; ignore or miss the bid and turn away; or push against the bid, igniting conflict. Gottman's research showed that couples who were happily together after six years and enjoying emotional and sexual connection turned towards each other's bids most of the time. Regular connections are therefore key and, critically, the attention we give each other has meaning beyond its content.

STRONG CONNECTIONS

Gottman's study (see below) showed the impact of responding to "bids for attention".

- ■ Couples who responded to attention 86% of the time stayed together happily.
- ▧ Couples who responded to attention just 33% of the time were least happy, or had split.

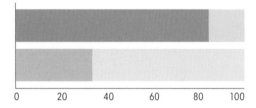

Is an unsatisfying sex life a deal breaker?

Whether or not problems with your sex life signal the end of a partnership will depend on the value and meaning each party places on sex within the relationship.

Sex is likely to cause challenges when those involved feel differently about it – for example, sex matters to one person and not the other, or when either or both partners don't want to work to address issues.

Sex can convey a great deal in relationships. Many of us feel that when sex is unsatisfactory or missing, or that a relationship is platonic, that it's hard to differentiate between this and a close friendship. Conversely, a lack of sex is less likely to be problematic for asexual people (see pp.36–37) or those with little or no interest in sex, who feel that there are more important components than sex to give a relationship value.

Dealing with problems

Where a satisfying sex life feels important, how we deal with issues when they arise can make a difference to whether or not we manage to overcome problems. If ongoing conflict about sex becomes a central theme of arguments, this is likely to lead to an accumulation of negative feelings and resentment, with partners feeling blame and frustration. This conflict and disruption can make you both less likely to have a potentially productive conversation, which could help you start to work together on ways to improve your sex life; in addition, conflict can leak out and disrupt other areas of your relationship.

OUR MOTIVES

Understanding each partner's motives for sex can highlight negative patterns; for example, having sex for the wrong reasons, such as fearing a partner will seek sex elsewhere. A willingness to resolve differences shows each party that they matter. Recognizing the need for change, and seeing if there's scope for improvement can be hugely beneficial for relationships.

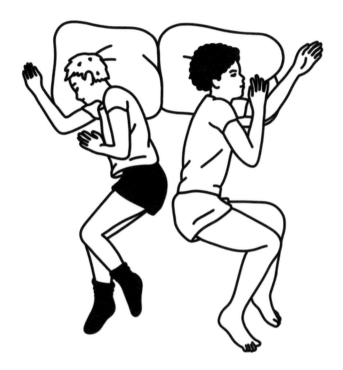

Different approaches

Where there's a discrepancy between what each partner desires, exploring ways to counter this can enable a relationship to continue, if wished. For example, if closeness and intimacy feel strong, but one partner requires more regular orgasms, pleasure, or a more active sex life, this is something that can be maintained through self-pleasure.

Some couples renegotiate their relationship style, opening it up to include sexual experiences with other partners as a way of navigating sexual differences. Moving into non-monogamous relationships (see p.30) takes consideration, communication, agreements, and negotiations. While for some couples this is the wrong approach, for others, opening up a relationship allows them to focus on the parts of their relationship that are working and positive; for them, rewriting their relationship rules and breaking away from a monogamous model can create the change they need.

Are **monogamy** and **fidelity** the same?

Humans are one of the few mammals that form monogamous bonds, but whether partnerships are faithful or not is dependent on the rules partners set for their relationship.

Monogamy is the relationship model of having only one sexual or romantic partner at one time, while fidelity is the choice to be faithful to someone. However, every couple co-writes their relationship rules, and within a monogamous relationship we can make choices, decisions, and agreements about what we want it to look like. Fidelity is about staying faithful to your partner within the agreement that you've made.

Relationship boundaries

Importantly, the agreements we make with partners shouldn't be assumed. Our relationship rules – akin to invisible contracts – are shaped by many factors, with different cultures having varying ideas about what's acceptable or not. This means that when we start an intimate relationship with someone, whatever the structure, we typically have guiding principles, rules, and ideas around what exclusivity will look like, and these may not align. For example, does one partner think that flirting or sexting (see opposite) doesn't count; or that a relationship can be "monogamish" (see p.31), with occasional sex outside a partnership acceptable?

While both may be happy with a definition, it can be helpful to explore your personal views of monogamy and fidelity at the start of a relationship, rather than assume you have the same ideas. By being explicit with each other, this ensures it's clear if one partner has violated the boundaries.

What's
sexting?

Sexting is a way to share elements of your sex life in a different dimension. It can build desire and anticipation, communicate to someone you're sexually aroused, or signal a desire for sex.

Sexting – the sharing of sexual content to a messaging format through phones and technology – may include text, voice notes, images, and videos. For those who find expressing themselves sexually in person difficult, the physical distance of sexting can help them open up. In one study of 1,265 US students, 50.1 per cent had sent an explicit text.

Safe sexting

Whether you're sexting a long-term or casual partner, it's important to protect yourself by agreeing that content is kept private. If you're concerned, keeping your face and identifying features, such as tattoos, out of shot can add a level of reassurance. If you share private or sexual images, you're giving consent at the time, but the consent doesn't extend beyond this exchange. Private and sexual content shared with the intention of causing distress and/ or without consent is termed image-based sexual abuse or revenge porn, which is illegal in the UK.

Is sexting cheating?

Whether sexting counts as cheating is dependent on the boundaries set in a relationship and whether you agree to allow non-physical connections that are sexual in nature. Although sexting doesn't involve sharing physical touch, it's a sexual exchange; if hidden from a partner, this can indicate a betrayal of trust.

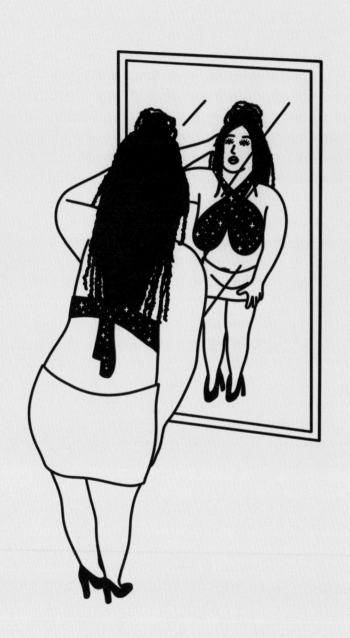

How can we rebuild sexual confidence after a breakup?

As we grow accustomed to a partner, initial feelings of self-consciousness fade and we start to feel safe. After a breakup, we need to re-engage the ability to take risks again.

Being in an intimate relationship carries the potential for emotional pain if it ends. Research shows that the stress of heartbreak increases levels of the stress hormone, cortisol. There's also a link between pain from social rejection and physical pain (see p.44). Our anxiety can make us cautious as we protect ourselves. In addition, we often hide social pain for fear of judgment, feeding a self-belief that we should get over an ex quickly.

Removing pressure

Feeling ready to have sex with someone new is completely subjective. For some, a period of separation that disassociates the topic of sex from a previous partner is helpful. Others feel ready to take a leap sooner. Part of the fear of trying something new is that the outcome is unknown; how willing we are to take a risk can depend on our psychological makeup and willingness to step out of comfort zones (see p.188). The key thing is to not pile pressure on ourselves to feel a certain way, which can create a sense we're acting because we don't feel genuinely ready.

It can be helpful to recognize that anxiety and excitement can manifest in a similar way. Physiologically, both increase the heart rate and trigger an adrenaline rush, or "butterflies". Anticipation also offers us a hit of the reward neurochemical dopamine (see p.56). This response is part of trying something new.

Self-nurturing time

Spending time with family and friends after a breakup can boost confidence and self-esteem as these interactions feed us socially and emotionally, helping us recalibrate. This also helps us think about our motivations for moving on and whether we're influenced by our couple-centric culture that suggests a relationship is needed to feel validated and valued.

When single, focusing on our sexual relationship with ourselves can be nurturing and refamiliarizes us with our sexual body; this can help us feel more confident when we decide we're ready for a partnered experience again.

Does sex **change** over time in relationships?

Rather than thinking about a relationship as stationary and linear, it can be more useful to view it as several different relationships with the same person over a period of time.

SEX IN LONG-TERM RELATIONSHIPS

A recent Mumsnet and Gransnet poll of 2,500 women, in association with Relate, looked at attitudes to sex within long-term relationships.

▨ 75% had satisfying relationship sex.
▨ 52% wanted more sex in their relationship.

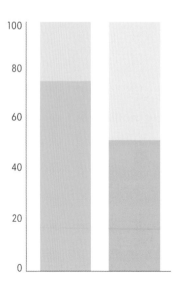

The most commonly reported experience is that sex declines in line with the length of a relationship. For many, though, less sex isn't necessarily a negative. Many in long-term relationships report sexual satisfaction in terms of feeling comfortable, confident, and intimate with their partner, contributing to higher levels of openness and communication, which can lead to more satisfying sex.

Can sexless relationships last?

There's no strict definition of a "sexless" relationship, especially as this often measures intercourse alone. Informally, a relationship is termed sexless if there's sexual activity less than 10 times a year or less than once a month. However, this suggests that our sex lives are objectively measurable. Asexual couples can have good relationships without sex, and some people have close intimate relationships with occasional sex. Others have periods of mental or physical ill health where sex is a lower priority. It's key to acknowledge that our sex lives go through changes, stages, and phases.

Can long-distance sex work?

Sex is definitely possible in a long-distance relationship, but partners may need to redefine what sex means to each of them.

To make sex work when you're separated by distance for significant periods of time, couples need to think about what sex will look like for them. Physical intimacy with a partner is of course heavily impacted in long-distance relationships. This can mean that scheduling in times (see p.182) to enjoy physical intimacy when possible may start to play a more dominant role, rather than relying on limited opportunities to be together to arise.

Embracing virtual sex

Typically, sex lives shift from being predominantly in-person to the virtual realm (see opposite) in long-distance relationships. There are plenty of virtual options to help keep desire alive when apart, incorporating a partner into your pleasure even if they're not physically present. With clear communication and boundaries, virtual sex can mean that distance doesn't have to signal an end to your sex life.

WHAT CAN VIRTUAL SEX INVOLVE?

Phone or video sex, sexting, and email messaging can become primary vehicles for sexual communication in long-distance relationships. Some couples also use teledildonics – sex toys that can be synced via the internet. Partners have toys with corresponding motions and sensations so that both parties experience simultaneous matching sensations; these can be used together with phone or video sex or sexting, extending human sexual interactions during virtual sex.

Working out boundaries that make you feel safe and comfortable can stop anxiety interfering with your ability to feel aroused or turned on during virtual sex. Privacy can be a key preoccupation or distraction. Some find it easier to relax and focus when they aren't watching themselves, so video sex may be a low priority or used with their screen off; for others, being able to see themselves feels arousing.

When will I be ready for postnatal sex?

While there are no fixed rules about when you can start having sex again, factors such as stitches and other bodily changes can mean it's advisable to wait at least a few weeks.

The decision to re-engage with sex after giving birth is best based around when you feel physically and emotionally ready. The early weeks with a baby can feel overwhelming as you grapple with sleep deprivation and hormonal changes, so it's not uncommon to deprioritize sex for a while. After birth, it's best not to focus on getting your sex life back to where it was, but to approach it in terms of what's best for you now.

It's possible to get pregnant again within three weeks of giving birth, even if you're breastfeeding and/or your periods haven't restarted, so thinking about contraception ahead of sex is an important consideration.

What's happening to your body?

Irrespective of whether you had a vaginal or Caesarean delivery, you'll have vaginal bleeding after birth; known as lochia, this comprises blood, mucus, and uterine tissue. It can last a few weeks so you may prefer to wait for this to stop before resuming sex.

Significant physical and hormonal changes during pregnancy, delivery, and after birth can change how you feel about your body at this time, and may affect when you feel like sex. Following a vaginal birth, the vaginal canal has a period of recovery after stretching to allow the baby to pass through, so you may want to wait until you feel more comfortable before having sex. If you needed an episiotomy – a cut made between the vagina and anus to facilitate delivery – it's advised to wait for the stitches to heal before engaging in penetrative sex.

Breastfeeding means that you have higher levels of prolactin, which suppresses ovulation and decreases oestrogen. Lower oestrogen when breastfeeding can cause vaginal dryness, which can make sex more painful, so lubricant is recommended.

Clear communication

Many people are concerned about sex feeling painful or different postnatally, and partners can also worry about causing pain. Physically, only you know how you feel, so communication, taking your time, and making space for reconnecting physically is critical. If intercourse is painful or uncomfortable, prioritizing non-penetrative

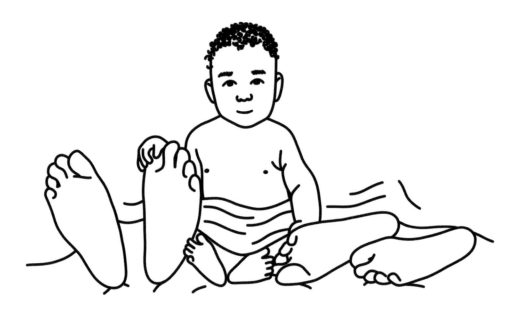

sexual contact can help you both still feel sexually connected. You may also want to set new boundaries temporarily. For example, some who previously enjoyed their breasts being touched feel that they don't provide the same pleasure while breastfeeding.

Studies show that male partners experience a permanent drop in testosterone after the birth of their baby. Evolutionary anthropologists, such as UK academic Dr Anna Machin, describe the impact this has on certain behaviours, such as a drop in libido and reduced aggression, as part of the evolutionary theory of "investing fathers" during this time.

Whatever your route to parenthood, becoming a parent marks a time of transition.

How do our genitals age?

Our entire body – including our genitals – goes through the ageing process. This doesn't mean, though, that we can't continue to enjoy a satisfying sex life.

As we age, our skin loses elasticity because of a reduction in the production of the proteins collagen and elastin, which give skin elasticity, keeping it supple and firm. As levels decrease, wrinkles form and skin starts to hang more loosely. This, together with hormonal changes and natural ageing processes, can age our genitals and affect function in line with the rest of our body.

- **Reduced collagen and elastin** thins tissues in the vulva; the labia may become less plump; and the scrotum may sag more.
- **A decline in oestrogen and testosterone** with age can lead to vaginal atrophy – the thinning, drying, and inflammation of the vaginal walls – which can make sex painful and uncomfortable. Vaginal atrophy can also affect those assigned female at birth (AFAB) trans people of any age taking testosterone. Painful sex can quickly

negatively reinforce sex as something we don't want to do, impacting desire and relationships. Using lubricant and vaginal moisturizers can be key to allow you to continue enjoying sex and penetration.
- **Pubic and body hair**, like the hair on our heads, changes with age. It starts to thin and can also go grey as production of melanin – the molecules that control pigmentation in our skin, hair, and eyes – slows down.

Reduced circulation

Numerous factors impact blood circulation as we get older, such as hypertension, which can lead to a hardening of blood vessels and reduced blood flow. This in turn can affect how our genitals feel and function. A reduced blood flow can impact sexual arousal (see p.93). When blood flow to the genitals decreases, this can affect the oxygenation of tissues

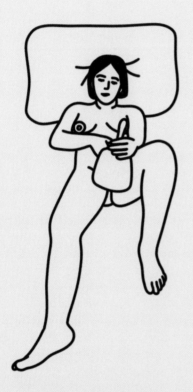

and may impact sensitivity. As a result, it may take more time and increased stimulation to reach previous levels of arousal and pleasure and we may need to adapt sexual routines, for example, by using lubricant or taking the emphasis off intercourse.

The effects of muscle decline

Muscle tone and mass is also lost with age, known as sarcopenia. A decline in muscle mass can impact the pelvic floor muscles, affecting the strength, intensity, and regularity of orgasms. For those with a penis, this can be associated with a reduction in ejaculation, as the pelvic floor muscles play a key role in ejecting semen. For all sexes, practising pelvic floor exercises (see p.112) can help you maintain this important hammock of muscles. Loss of muscle tone can also contribute to scrotal sagging.

As with the rest of our lives, our bodies go through phases and stages.

Does **menopause** affect sex?

While symptoms may impact your sex life, menopause certainly doesn't have to mean the end of sex. There are plenty of ways to ensure pleasure and sexual wellbeing endure.

Perimenopause and menopause are brought on by the natural decline in the hormones oestrogen, progesterone, and testosterone that occurs with ageing. Menopause is defined as not having had a period for 12 months, marking the end of ovulation and fertility. Menopause usually occurs naturally, but can be induced medically, for example, after surgery to remove the ovaries, or after treatments such as radiation or chemotherapy. Rarely, premature ovarian insufficiency can cause a rapid onset of symptoms.

Menopause isn't just something that cisgender women experience; those who are

Menopause signals a period of physical, emotional, and psychological change.

non-binary, intersex, and trans men can go through the menopause. However, hormonal treatments and/or surgical interventions may change someone's menopausal experience.

How can symptoms affect us?

There are around 34 common symptoms of menopause, including anxiety, vaginal dryness, mood changes, hot flushes, brain fog, interrupted sleep, and reduced libido. Most experience some symptoms, which can influence many areas of wellbeing, including sleep, cognitive function, and sex.

Menopause can influence our sex lives in a variety of ways. Lower levels of oestrogen lead to vaginal dryness, one of the most common menopausal symptoms, which can make penetrative sex difficult and uncomfortable. Reduced oestrogen and testosterone can also impact our interest in sex, with a lack of desire and difficulty becoming aroused commonly reported. Other symptoms such as fatigue, hot flushes, and anxiety can affect our motivation for sex. It's important to discuss changes with partners so they understand what does feel good and is possible for you in terms of your sex life and pleasure. Otherwise, repeatedly doing something that isn't working for you can lead to a negative relationship with sex, further impacting desire.

Making menopause work

Lifestyle adjustments that help maximize health and wellbeing can help you manage symptoms. For some, hormone replacement therapy (HRT), taken under the guidance of a healthcare provider, is helpful. This supplies oestrogen and progestogen, relieving symptoms such as vaginal dryness, mood swings, and hot flushes – topical oestrogen is also available for vaginal dryness. Medical practitioners can also offer testosterone on a case-by-case basis.

While many find menopause challenging, for others it can feel liberating. Freed from monthly periods – especially welcome where cycles were painful or problematic – and pregnancy worries, once past perimenopause, they may find renewed motivation for sex.

WHAT'S THE ANDROPAUSE?

The term andropause, or "male menopause", can be misleading as this isn't a distinct transitional stage associated with the end of fertility. However, for cis men in their 40s and 50s, the gradual decline in testosterone – that occurs at a rate of about 1–2 per cent a year after the age of 30 – can start to affect mood and energy levels. If you're concerned about your testosterone levels, these can be checked with a blood test, ideally done in the mornings when levels peak.

How can we keep the conversation going?

Creating a positive relationship with sex throughout our lives can help us shape our sensual world and enjoy fulfilling sexual relationships.

Normalizing sex involves moving away from negative messaging about what sex should be about and moving towards our authentic sexual selves. This doesn't mean we have to bare all and unpack our sex lives publicly, but that we feel we have freedom and choice to do what we want with them. We're able to let go of self-judgment and judgment of others. The fundamental principles below can guide you to a greater understanding of how sex can be positioned in your life.

1

Understand that sex can be different things to different people. As long as it's consensual and legal, we can try to accept each other's differences and that we're not all perfectly aligned. Acceptance doesn't have to be agreement, but simply an acknowledgment of diversity.

2

Communication is a huge part of navigating and accepting differences and is the source of understanding between us. Without communicating, we can only guess what others think, and feelings of shame can arise.

IS IT JUST ME WHO STRUGGLES WITH SEX?

Questions on sex are one of the most searched items online, and numerous brands promote products to help our sex lives – sex is profitable because people want help. Challenges are common, but talking about problems isn't; the irony is that talking would be a large part of the solution as so many challenges are psychological, set up by social expectations.

One of the most common side effects of struggling with sex is feeling isolated. Finding a trusted person to talk to – whether a partner, family member, friend, or professional – can help us face sources of anxiety rather than avoid them. In turn, we can learn and rebuild a model of sex that suits us better.

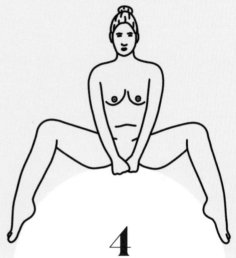

4
Connecting with ourselves physically – owning our pleasure – boosts our sexual confidence and builds a positive relationship with ourselves, our desires, and our sensuality.

3
By listening, we become more sexually aware. We notice the language and narratives around us and can challenge ideas about sex we feel don't work for us. Listening to others also helps us examine our own ideas about sex through a wide-angle lens, broadening our perspective.

How do I keep sex
relevant?

We have the best sex when we break away from preconceived notions and decide ourselves what good sex looks like for us. This self-awareness is at the core of maintaining our sexual wellbeing.

Shape your own sexual culture

As individuals, we're partly defined by the context of what's going on around us in the world, whether economical, political, and/or cultural. To some degree these contexts shape our lives and, ultimately, the sex we might have.

Much change is needed to society's approach to sex. However, bringing about large-scale change takes time. While we wait for broader societal change to happen, we can work to ensure we're happy with our own relationship with sex. Throughout our lives, we hold onto things we value and let go of what no longer holds importance. Applying this approach to our sex lives can help us shape our own sexual culture so we change our relationship with sex for the better. This in turn can create a ripple effect as we start to challenge the norms and redesign our sexual narratives.

Prioritize sexual wellbeing

Placing our sexual wellbeing alongside other areas of our health and not treating it as an afterthought elevates your sex life to where it deserves to be. Many find communicating

their sexual needs one of the hardest things to do, but it's one of the most effective tools for enhancing our sex lives and is the only way that we can really expect to be understood, or for us to understand others.

Maintain sexual self-awareness

Developing our sexual self-awareness is about recognizing what we need and when, whether that be pressing pause on our sex lives, or leaning into exploring something new. Keep in mind that the basic premise of the sex we have is about consensually giving and receiving pleasure; how we achieve that might change throughout different periods of our lives, based on our motivations, health, relationships, and sense of self. Breaking away mentally from a shaming sexual culture allows us to redesign our sex lives, personalizing them to allow us to achieve our sexual potential.

The healthiest
relationship with
our sexual selves is
one disconnected
from shame.

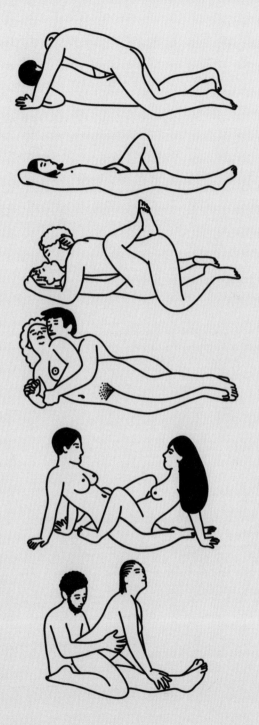

Glossary

Aphrodisiacs Substances commonly found in foods that are believed to increase attraction, desire, pleasure, and sexual behaviours.

Aromantic/Aromanticism Refers to someone who experiences little or no romantic attraction to, or interest in, others.

Arousal *See Sexual arousal.*

Arousal non-concordance The disconnect between a person's physical and psychological and/or emotional experience of arousal, where the body and mind are out of sync. For example, a person may feel psychologically turned on, but struggle to experience physical arousal; or they may feel physically aroused, but unable to emotionally connect with their *sexual arousal*.

Asexuality In the sexual orientation spectrum, this describes someone who experiences no or low sexual attraction to others, and/or someone who has little or no interest in sexual experiences and/ or behaviours. Someone can be described as asexual or an asexual person.

Assigned male at birth (AMAB)/Assigned female at birth (AFAB) Refers to the label that a medical professional assigns a baby when it's born, based on external physical anatomy.

BDSM An abbreviation for bondage, discipline (or domination), sadism (or submission), masochism. BDSM is an umbrella term for a range of consensual practices commonly involving role play, exchanges of control, power, and intense sensory stimulation.

Bids for attention A bid from one partner to another in an attempt to get their affection, attention, or positive connection. Famously researched in couples by Dr John Gottman.

Biopsychosocial approach Examines the interaction between biological, psychological, and socio-environmental factors in terms of understanding our health and wellbeing.

Body confidence How a person feels about their body and the way they look.

Body dysmorphia/Body dysmorphic disorder (BDD) A mental health condition where someone spends a lot of time and attention worrying and focusing on perceived flaws in their appearance. The perceived flaws are often not apparent to other people.

Body neutrality The approach to accepting and appreciating our bodies without the demand or pressure to love them. It's guided by principles of respect and focusing on how our bodies feel rather than how they look.

Body positivity An encompassing term for celebrating body diversity and all bodies. It encourages body appreciation, love, and confidence and challenges societal and popular messages about body "norms", which can influence a person's body image.

Butt plug A sex toy that's designed to be inserted into the anus for sexual pleasure and stimulation. It is also used to help relax the anal sphincter in preparation for penetration. Anal toys should always have a flared base for safe use.

Cisgender Someone whose gender identity aligns with the sex they were assigned at birth. *See also Gender identity.*

Cock ring A ring usually worn around the base of the penis to produce stronger erections, or maintain erections for longer. It works by physically restricting blood flow, trapping blood in the penis. Numerous versions are available.

Cognitive Our cognition is a brain function that relates to our conscious mental activities, such as thinking, learning, remembering, and reasoning.

Consent The ongoing process of agreement between all participants to engage in sexual activity, which has to be freely and clearly communicated without coercion.

Contraception Also known as birth control or fertility control, contraception is the deliberate use of various methods or techniques to prevent pregnancy as a consequence of sexual intercourse. Options include barrier methods, such as condoms, the cap, and diaphragm; hormonal methods, such as the contraceptive pill and hormonal intrauterine system (IUS), or coil; or the non-hormonal, copper intrauterine device (IUD); as well as sterilization procedures and natural family planning/fertility awareness techniques. Barrier methods can also be used to prevent transmission of *sexually transmitted infections (STIs)*.

Cortisol The body's primary stress hormone, produced by the adrenal glands.

Cum Commonly used term for *orgasm* and/or ejaculate or *ejaculation*.

Dental dam A square piece of stretchy latex that is worn over the vulva or anus during oral sex to help prevent the spread of *sexually transmitted infections (STIs)*.

Desire A person's want and motivation for a sexual experience. It can either be *spontaneous*, when desire happens seemingly out of the blue and occurs in anticipation of a sexual experience; or desire can be *responsive*, which can be thought of as the desire to continue with sex, as desire emerges in response to sexual stimulation.

Dildo A sex toy that most commonly resembles a shape similar to an erect penis, usually used for penetrative stimulation.

Dopamine A neurotransmitter that plays a crucial role in the functioning of the body and the brain, and a key role in the brain's reward system and our experiences of pleasure.

Dual-control model A model that frames sexual response as a balance between inhibitory and excitatory processes, where each individual has their own level of inhibitory and excitatory sensitivity.

Ejaculation The ejection of semen from the body through the penis, commonly – but not exclusively – paired with *orgasm*.

Endorphins Brain chemicals that are released to help us cope with the perception of pain and stress and which can also lift mood. They're released when we experience pain, stress, and pleasure, and during activities such as sex, exercise, and massage, which explains scenarios such as "a runner's high".

Erectile dysfunction When a person is unable to achieve or maintain a penile erection, potentially interrupting their ability to have certain sexual experiences, such as penetrative sex.

Erection The hardening of the penis. This occurs when spongy tissue in the penis shaft, known as the corpora cavernosa, relaxes and blood flows in, creating pressure that traps the blood, making the penis harden and stand away from the body. Erections can be *reflexogenic*, in response to direct stimulation of the penis; or *psychogenic*, when the brain has sexual thoughts. While erections happen mostly during sexual arousal, they can also occur during sleep, known as nocturnal erections.

Erogenous zone A sensitive spot on the body that can increase sexual feelings, and/or desire when touched. Extragenital erogenous zones are ones that don't involve the genitals, for example, the nipples, neck, and ears.

Erotic Something that triggers sexual desire, interest, arousal, or excitement. Some materials, such as erotic literature and audio erotica, are specifically designed to arouse. What we find erotic is highly subjective.

Ethical/Consensual non-monogamy The relationship practice of having sexual and/or intimate relationships with more than one partner. Importantly, this carries the consent of all parties involved. Non-monogamous relationships can take many different forms as agreed between partners.

Fetish An object or non-genital body part that's strongly linked to sexual arousal, desire, and/or gratification. The person who has the fetish is called a fetishist.

Foreplay A common term for non-penetrative sex in preparation for intercourse. However, this terminology denotes an order of sex, indicating that these experiences come "before" penetrative sex, which isn't preferable to everyone. For some people, therefore, reframing foreplay as *non-penetrative sex* can be helpful.

G spot The Gräfenberg "spot" is a highly sensitive area or zone located a few centimetres into the vagina on the anterior wall. Forming part of the clitoral network, it can swell during sexual arousal and provide pleasure from stimulation.

Gender binary The classification of gender into two distinct categories, male and female. *See also* non-binary.

Gender dysphoria A term used to describe the sense of unease and/or psychological distress a person may have due to a mismatch between their *gender identity* and the sex they were assigned at birth.

Genderfluid Describes someone who has a non-fixed gender identity, who does not identify as having a single or unchanging gender.

Gender identity Each person's individual and internal experience of their gender.

Gender-affirming care As defined by the WHO, this encompasses a range of social, psychological, behavioural, and medical interventions "designed to support and affirm an individual's gender identity".

Genitals The body's external sexual and reproductive organs. Comprises the penis, scrotum, and the vulva, which includes the vaginal opening.

Habituation The reduction in behavioural response to a repeated stimulus This is a type of non-associative learning, meaning that there's no punishment or reward associated to the stimulus.

Heteronormative The concept and assumption that heterosexuality is considered the normal or preferred mode of sexual orientation; a part of this is that heterosexuality is often privileged over other sexual orientations.

Hormones See *Sex hormones.*

Intercourse The sexual experience that typically involves penetrative sex, with a penis being inserted into a vagina. Also called sexual intercourse; *PIV sex*

(penis-in-vagina penetration); penetrative sex; vaginal intercourse; and vaginal sex.

Intersex An umbrella term for people with a biological diversity of chromosomes, reproductive organs, genitals, or hormones that fall outside the typical binary of male/female biology. Intersex characteristics are a naturally occurring variation in humans.

Intimacy The dynamic and closeness of an interpersonal relationship. Intimacy and sex can be closely linked for some people, but they aren't synonymous. Intimacy doesn't have to be sexual or take place in a sexual or partnered relationship. It can be emotional or physical; for example, we can have deep intimacy with family or friends.

Intimacy coordinator A professional who specializes in coordinating and choreographing simulated sex and intimacy scenes in film, TV, and theatre productions; protecting the wellbeing of those involved in these scenes.

Kink A broad term for consensual sexual activities that are often considered unconventional and unusual. Someone may be described as kinky. The terms may be used comparatively as the opposite of more traditional "vanilla sex".

Labiaplasty The surgical procedure to reduce or alter the size of the labia minora.

Libido Commonly referred to as sex drive, this describes our sexual instincts, drive, and desire for sex and pleasure. Influenced by biological, social, and psychological factors, we can see fluctuations and changes to libido throughout our lives. There's no standardized baseline or level for libido and it varies from person to person.

Lubricant A sexual aid, typically a liquid or gel, that's applied to the genitals, anus, or products such as sex toys or dilators, to reduce friction between body parts, making penetration easier and experiences more comfortable and pleasurable.

Make-up sex A colloquial term for sex after conflict, typically in an intimate or partnered relationship.

Masturbation The self-stimulation of the genitals for pleasure, most often using hands or sex toys.

Also known as self-pleasure, solo sex, and numerous other conversational terms.

Metacognition The process of thinking about our thinking, often referring to the way we try to assess our own performance or understanding.

Metoidioplasty The gender-affirming, lower body surgery/s to create a penis from the existing genitalia – that is, the vaginal tissue and clitoris.

Mindful sex Mindfulness is the practice of purposely bringing our attention to our in-the-moment, present experience, without passing judgment or evaluation. In the context of sex, this is the conscious practice of directing our attention non-judgementally to the present moment and what we're experiencing sensually.

Mononormative The often unconscious assumption that relationships that are monogamous are the norm, or used as a measure or standard; this can privilege monogamy over other relationship structures.

Neurodivergent The term used to describe an individual who has a brain that works differently from someone who is neurotypical.

Neurodiversity The term used to describe the variability in all human brains and cognition, and the unique ways that different people's brains work.

Neuroplasticity Also known as neural plasticity or brain plasticity, this is the ability of neural networks in the brain to grow and change with learning, sometimes described as the idea of "the brain that changes itself".

Neurotransmitters The body's essential chemical messengers that travel between cells and are associated with specific bodily reactions and responses.

Non-binary An umbrella term for those who don't identify within the gender binary.

Non-penetrative sex This describes physical sexual experiences that don't involve penetration (with a penis or sex toy). Also described as *outercourse* or *foreplay*.

Orgasm A peak brain and body pleasure experience, characterized by a build up and release of muscular tension and neurochemical release. Most often associated with stimulation of the genitals, but can be achieved by other means.

Outercourse Describes non-penetrative sexual experiences. Used as an alternative word for *foreplay*, to avoid implying a set order to sex.

Oxytocin A neurochemical that plays a critical role in sex, childbirth, breastfeeding, and social interactions, and in bonding behaviours.

PDE5 inhibitors Stands for "phosphodiesterase type 5" inhibitors; medications that improve blood flow to certain tissues, commonly used to treat erectile dysfunction. They include Viagra (Sildenafil), Cialis (tadalafil), Levitra (vardenafil), and Stendra (avanafil).

PEP Standing for "post-exposure prophylaxis", this is an HIV medication that can stop HIV infection taking hold after the virus enters the body. It must be taken within 72 hours of possible exposure, ideally as soon as possible.

Performance anxiety When specifically in relation to sex, this is the apprehension or anxiety about a sexual experience, often when it's goal-orientated, which creates pressure and distraction. Most commonly, it's described by people with penises having anxiety and/or related erection difficulties.

Phalloplasty The surgical procedure/s to construct or reconstruct a penis, commonly using areas of skin from other parts of the body.

Pheromones Chemicals secreted by animals to trigger a social response in members of the same species.

Physiological The science of how the body functions, including the chemistry and physics of how the structures of the body work.

PIV sex Stands for "penis-in-vagina" penetration. Also known as *intercourse* or penetrative sex.

Polyamory Describes engaging in romantic and/or sexual relationships with more than one person at the same time, with the informed consent of all partners involved. An example of *Ethical or consensual non-monogamy*.

Pornography Material, usually film or print but can be audio, containing explicit descriptions and/or depictions of sexual content. Designed to arouse and elicit sexual excitement.

PrEP Standing for "pre-exposure prophylaxis", this is a drug taken before and after sex by HIV-negative people to reduce their risk of getting HIV.

Pre-cum Also known as pre-ejaculate, this is a small amount of fluid that's involuntarily released from the penis during arousal, usually separate and before ejaculation, hence the name.

Prostate gland A gland located below the bladder and in front of the rectum in those assigned male at birth. It plays a part in reproduction, and can be stimulated for pleasure via the perineum and/or anus.

Psychogenic erection A reaction that originates in the mind; for example, an erection that occurs in response to sexual thoughts.

Psychosexual therapy Also known as psychosexual counselling, and sometimes sex therapy, this is a talking therapy specifically focusing on sexual difficulties, challenges, or concerns.

Psychosomatic The interaction between the mind and body. It's often used to describe symptoms that may be rooted in psychology and emotions without any other clear physical explanation.

Reflexogenic A reaction caused by a reflex, for example an erection that results from direct touch or stimulation of the penis.

Refractory period The time or recovery period after an orgasm when a person temporarily isn't sexually responsive.

Responsive desire The desire for sex or a sexual experience that emerges in response to sexual stimulation. It's different to *spontaneous desire*, which arises in anticipation of a sexual experience.

Revenge porn The sharing and distribution of sexually explicit videos or images of a person without their consent, with the intent to cause distress. Importantly, videos or photos may have been recorded between partners with consent at the time, but this consent cannot be applied to the sharing of this content. In the UK, revenge pornography is a criminal offence.

Sex hormones The main hormones that play an instrumental role in reproduction and fertility, sexual response, and sexual development. The main reproductive and sex hormones are oestrogen, progesterone, and testosterone.

Sex toy An object specifically designed to give and be used for sexual pleasure.

Sexology The interdisciplinary study of human sexual behaviour. A sexologist is a person who studies human sexual behaviour.

Sexting Sharing sexual content via direct or personal messages, such as on a mobile phone or via social media messaging.

Sexual arousal The physiological and psychological responses to sexual stimuli or stimulation that act to prepare the body for a sexual experience.

Sexual concordance Refers to the degree that our physical and genital arousal corresponds to our psychological and subjective (self-reported) *sexual arousal*. The opposite term is sexual/*arousal non-concordance*.

Sexual currency The sexually charged connections and actions between partners that are building blocks within our sex lives, without in themselves being sex. For example, extended hugs, lingering kisses, or flirting.

Sexual dysfunction Characterized by recurring and/or persistent problems with sexual response and functioning, including sexual pain and problems with desire, arousal, and orgasm.

Sexual orientation The emotional, sexual, or romantic attraction that a person feels towards another person or others. Examples include bisexual, gay, lesbian, heterosexual, pansexual, and asexual.

Sexuality An individual's sense of being a sexual being. This can include attitudes, thoughts, beliefs, desires, behaviours, as well as identity related to sex.

Sexually transmitted infections (STIs) Infections that are predominantly spread through sex, particularly unprotected sex. Common infections include chlamydia, gonorrhoea, trichomoniasis, and syphilis. Many infections are asymptomatic, highlighting the importance of sexual health screening to confirm a person's status.

Spontaneous desire An interest or motivation for sex that seemingly arises out of the blue, in anticipation of a sexual experience.

Squirting The conversational term for the expulsion of liquid during an orgasm or intense pleasure that some people with vulvas experience.

Strap-on Worn usually with a harness around the hips in the usual position of a penis, a strap-on is a dildo or sex toy worn against the body rather than manually held.

Swinging The practice of couples or partners engaging in group sex or partner-swapping sexual experiences, with the consent and agreement of all of those involved.

Tantric sex A sexual practice that's part of the ancient spiritual path, tantra. It focuses on the bringing together of sexuality and spirituality, with an emphasis on intimacy and connection, rather than a goal-orientated model of sex.

Tenting The process that the vagina goes through during sexual arousal and excitement. The uterus pulls up and the vagina expands to create more space for comfortable penetration.

Trans The umbrella term to describe people whose *gender identity* doesn't align with the sex that they were assigned at birth.

Transitioning The gender-affirming process of making changes so that you can live in your *gender identity*. Transitioning can be social, medical (hormonal), or surgical, or any combination of these.

Vaginal atrophy The thinning, drying, and inflammation of the vaginal walls. Most commonly related to hormonal changes, for example, as a result of menopause.

Vaginal dilators A set of tube-shaped products that come in increasing sizes to stretch the vagina, for example after *vaginoplasty* procedures or as treatment for certain gynaecological cancers; or to train the pelvic floor muscles to enable vaginal penetration in painful sex conditions such as *vaginismus* and dyspareunia.

Vaginismus A condition characterized by the involuntary tightening of the group of muscles, known as the pelvic floor muscles, around the vagina when penetration is attempted.

Vaginoplasty A surgical procedure to construct or repair the vagina.

Vibrator A type of *sex toy* with vibration settings to produce pleasurable sensations and sexual stimulation.

Virtual sex The phenomenon of technology-mediated sexual interactions or experiences, rather than being physically together in person. It can also be called cyber sex, and can include video sex, *sexting*, and using teledildonics.

Vulva External *genitals* that comprises the vagina and urethral openings, the labia minora and majora, the mons pubis, and glans clitoris.

Vulvodynia Persistent, unexplained pain and discomfort in the vulva that can't be explained by any other identifiable cause.

Bibliography

All website links accessed March 2023.

11 A brief history of sex
Imperial College London (2019). [online]. By 2037 half of babies likely to be born to couples who met online. www.imperial.ac.uk/news/194152

16-17 Sex good for your health
Ditzen, B. et al. (2019). Intimacy as related to cortisol reactivity and recovery in couples undergoing psychosocial stress. *Psychosom Med.* 81(1). 16-25. DOI: 10.1097/01.psy.0000552769.11461.31
Murray, S. H. and Brotto, L. (2021). I want you to want me: a qualitative analysis of heterosexual men's desire to feel desired in intimate relationships. *J. Sex Marital Ther* [online]. 47 (5). 419-34. DOI.org/10.1080/0092623X.2021.1888830

22-23 What happens when we think about sex?
Educare. What is metacognition? (2020). [online] www.educare.co.uk/news/what-is-metacognition

26-27 Solo sex
Hurlbert, D. F. (1991). The role of masturbation in marital and sexual satisfaction: a comparative study of female masturbators and nonmasturbators. *J Sex Educ Ther.* 17 (4). 272-82. DOI.10.1080/01614576.1991.11074029
Corrigan, F. M. (2014). Shame and the vestigial midbrain urge to withdraw. Neurobiology and treatment of traumatic dissociation. DOI: 10.1891/9780826106322.0009
The Monkey Therapist. [online] https://themonkeytherapist.com

32-33 Sex and shame
Davis, S. (2019). The neuroscience of shame. CPTSD foundation. [online]. https://cptsdfoundation.org/2019/04/11/the-neuroscience-of-shame/

34-35 Sex and intimacy
Rocco, S. C. (2019). Neuroanatomy and function of human sexual behaviour: A neglected or unknown issue? Brain and Behavior [online]. 9 (12). E01389. www.ncbi.nlm.nih.gov/pmc/articles/PMC6908863/

38 Can we get better at sex?
Warrell, M. (2015). Use it or lose it: The science behind self-confidence. *Forbes.* [online]. www.forbes.com/sites/margiewarrell/2015/02/26/build-self-confidence-5strategies

42-43 Does context change sex?
Meston, C. M. and Buss, D.M. (2007). Why humans have sex. *Arch Sex Behav.* [online]. 36. 477-507. https://labs.la.utexas.edu/mestonlab/files/2016/05/WhyHaveSex.pdf
Nagoski, E. (2015). *Come as You Are.* UK: Scribe

44-45 Can I ask my partner to wait?
Wnuk, A. (2018). Do hurt feelings actually hurt? *Brain Facts.* [online]. www.brainfacts.org/thinking-sensing-and-behaving/emotions-stress-and-anxiety
Garland, E. L. (2012). Pain processing in the human nervous system. *Prim Care.* 39 (3). 561-71. DOI: 10.1016/j.pop.2012.06.013
Hayati, A. (2014). The brain in pain. *Malays J Med Sci.* 21 (Spec Issue). 46-54. PMC4405805

46-47 Are we having enough sex?
Mitchell, K. R. et al. (2013). Sexual function in Britain: findings from the third national survey of sexual attitudes and lifestyles (Natsal-3). *Lancet.* [online] 382. 1817-1829. www.natsal.ac.uk/sites/default/files/2021-04/Natsal-3%20infographics.pdf
Wolfinger, N. H. (2021). Is the sex recession turning into a great sex depression? *IF Studies.* [online]. https://ifstudies.org/blog/is-the-sex-recession-turning-into-a-great-sex-depression
The Australian Study of Health and Relationships [online] www.ashr.edu.au/

48-49 Will disability affect my sex life?
UK Legislation. Equality Act 2010. [online]. www.legislation.gov.uk/ukpga/2010/15/section/6?view=extent

50-51 Am I broken?
Mitchell, K. R. et al. (2013). Sexual function in Britain: findings from the third national survey of sexual attitudes and lifestyles (Natsal-3). *Lancet.* [online] 382. 1817-1829. www.natsal.ac.uk/sites/default/files/2021-04/Natsal-3%20infographics.pdf

52-53 Am I normal?
Simon, W. and Gagnon, J. H. (1986). Sexual scripts: permanence and change. *Arch Sex Behav.* 15. 97-120. DOI: 10.1007/BF01542219

54-55 Emotional vulnerability after sex
Schweitzer, R. D. (2015). Postcoital dysphoria: prevalence and psychological correlates. *Sex Med.* 3 (4). 235-43. DOI: 10.1002/sm2.74
Maczkowiack, J. and Schweitzer, R. (2019). Postcoital dysphoria: Prevalence and correlates among males. *J Sex Mar Ther.* 45 (2), 128-40. DOI: 10.1080/0092623X.2018.1488326
Bhardwaj, N. (2020). Is crying after sex normal? *Health Shots.* [online]. www.healthshots.com/intimate-health/sexual-health/is-crying-after-sex-normal-a-psychologist-answers/

56-57 What is pleasure?
Mcleod, S. (2023). Brain reward system. *Simply Psychology.* [online]. www.simplypsychology.org/brain-reward-system.html
Uniformed Services University of the Health Sciences (2017). How PTSD affects the brain. *Brainline.* [online]. www.brainline.org/article/how-ptsd-affects-brain

64-65 Can fantasies enhance sex?
Orwig, J. (2014). Scientists have discovered how common different sexual fantasies are. *Business Insider.* [online]. www.businessinsider.com/which-sexual-fantasies-are-normal-2014-10
Tseng, J. and Poppenk, J. (2020). Brain meta-state transitions demarcate thoughts across task contexts exposing the mental noise of trait neuroticism. *Nat Commun.* [online]. 11. 3480. DOI: 10.1038/s41467-020-17255-9
Lehmiller, J. (2018). *Tell Me What You Want: The Science of Sexual Desire and How It Can Help You Improve Your Sex Life.* Robinson.

68-69 Body knowledge
Intima (2020). 25% of women can't correctly identify vagina [online]. www.intimina.com/blog/women-and-their-bodies/
Sex Education Forum. (2022). Young People's RSE Poll 2021. [online]. www.sexeducationforum.org.uk/resources/evidence/young-peoples-rse-poll-2021

Ferguson, R. M. et al. (2008). A matter of facts and more: An exploratory analysis of the content of sexuality education in The Netherlands. *Sex Ed.* [online]. 8 (1). 93-106. DOI: 10.1080/14681810701811878

The Eve Appeal (2016). Why 'vagina' should be part of every young woman's vocabulary. [online]. https://eveappeal.org.uk/wp-content/uploads/2016/07/The-Eve-Appeal-Vagina-Dialogues.pdf

Reeves, L. (2021). My vulva and I. Lydia Reeves. [online]. www.lydiareeves.com/my-vulva-and-i

Henshaw, P. (2022). Relationships and sex education: Too many still not being taught the basics. *SecEd*. [online]. www.sec-ed.co.uk/news/relationships-and-sex-education-too-many-still-not-being-taught-the-basics

US adolescents' receipt of formal sex education. (2022). Guttmacher Institute. [online]. www.guttmacher.org/fact-sheet/adolescents-teens-receipt-sex-education-united-states

Nielsen-Bohlman, L. (2004). Health Literacy: A prescription to end confusion. *US: NAP*. DOI: 10.17226/10883

70-71 Am I normal?
Kalampalikis, A. and Michala, L. (2021). Cosmetic labiaplasty on minors: a review of current trends and evidence. *Int J Impot Res*. DOI: 10.1038/s41443-021-00480-1

Aleem, S. & Adams, E. J. (2012). Labiaplasty. *Obstet, Gynaecol Reprod Med*. 22 (2). 50-53. DOI: 10.1016/j.ogrm.2011.11.006

Turini, T. et al. The impact of labiaplasty on sexuality. *Plast Reconstr Surg*. 141 (1). 87-92. DOI: 10.1097/PRS.0000000000003921

72-73 Vagina or vulva?
Murphy, C. (2016). Sexperts say this is your most underrated erogenous zone - here's what to do it. *Women's Health* [online]. www.womenshealthmag.com/sex-and-love/a19946348/mons-pubis-sex-tips/

Science Direct. Mon Pubis. [online]. www.sciencedirect.com/topics/medicine-and-dentistry/mons-pubis

74-75 What happens to the vagina during sex?
Sullivan, C. and Jio, S. (2022). 21vagina facts that every person with one should know. *Woman's Day* [online]. www.womansday.com/health-fitness/womens-health/a5466/8-things-you-didnt-know-about-your-vagina-113565/

Ilyich, I. (2021). What's the difference between vaginal discharge, arousal fluid, and cervical mucus? *Flo* [online]. https://flo.health/menstrual-cycle/health/vaginal-discharge/discharge-fluid-mucus

76-77 The clitoris
Maravilla, K. et al. (2003). Dynamic MR imaging of the sexual arousal response in women', *J Sex Marital Ther*, 29: 71-6. DOI: 10.1080/713847132

El-Hamamsy, D. et al. (2022). Public understanding of female genital anatomy and pelvic organ prolapse (POP); a questionnaire-based pilot study. *Int Urogynecol J*. 33. 309-18. DOI: 10.1007/s00192-021-04727-9

Gross, R. E. The clitoris, uncovered: an intimate history. *Scientific American*. (2020) [online]. www.scientificamerican.com/article/the-clitoris-uncovered-an-intimate-history/

O'Connell, H. E. and Sanjeevan, K.V. (2005). Anatomy of the clitoris. *PubMed*. 174 (4). 1189-95. DOI: 10.1097/01.ju.0000173639.38898.cd

78-79 Male sex organs
National Cancer Institute. Penis. [online]. https://training.seer.cancer.gov/anatomy/reproductive/male/penis.html

80-81 Penis anxiety
Francken, A. B. et al. (2002). What importance do women attribute to the size of the penis? *Eur Urol*. 42 (5). 426-31. DOI: 10.1016/s0302-2838(02)00396-2

Tiggemann, M. et al. (2008). Beyond muscles: unexplored parts of men's body image. *J Health Psychol*. 13 (8). 1163-72. 10.1177/1359105308095971

GMFA. (2017). Penis anxiety is impacting gay men's self-esteem. *LGBT Hero*. [online]. www.lgbthero.org.uk/fs160-penis-anxiety-is-impacting-gay-mens-self-esteem

82-83 Transitioning
Tordoff, D. M. et al. (2022). Mental health outcomes in transgender and nonbinary youths receiving gender-affirming care. *JAMA Network Open*. 5 (2). E220978. DOI: 10.1001/jamanetworkopen.2022.0978

Stonewall. (2018). LGBT in Britain - Health (online). www. https://stonewall.org.uk/lgbt-britain-health

84-85 The G spot
Vieira-Baptista, P. et al. (2021). G-spot: fact or fiction?. *Sex Med*. 9 (5). 100435. DOI: 10.1016/j.esxm.2021.100435

National Women's Health Network (2022). Is the G-spot real? *NWHN*. [online]. https://nwhn.org/is-the-g-spot-real/

Puppo, V. (2012). Does the G-spot exist? *Int Urogynecol J*. 23 (12). 1665-9. DOI: 10.1007/s00192-012-1831-y

Psychology Today (2009). The most important sexual statistic [online]. www.psychologytoday.com/us/blog/all-about-sex/200903/the-most-important-sexual-statistic

86-87 Using lube/genital hygiene
Bloom Ob/Gyn (2018). Vaginal Hygiene - Do's and Dont's. [online]. https://bloom-obgyn.com/vaginal-hygiene-dos-and-donts/

88-89 What happens in brain when touched?
App, B. et al. (2006). Touch communicates distinct emotions. *American Psychological Association*. [online] 6 (3). 528-33. https://citeseerx.ist.psu.edu/viewdoc/download?doi=10.1.1.421.2391&rep=rep1&type=pdf

Wired (2017). The science of touch. [online] www.wired.co.uk/article/the-good-life-human-touch

Michels, L. et al (2010). The somatosensory representation of the human clitoris: an fMRI study, *NeuroImage* 49 (1). 177-84. DOI: 10.1016/j.neuroimage.2009.07.024

Crichon, P. (1994). Penfield's homunculus. *J Neurol Neurosurg Psychiatry*. 57 (525). Published Online First: 01 Apr 1994. DOI: 10.1136/jnnp.57.4.525

90-91 Erogenous zones
Nummenmaa, L. et al. (2016). Topography of human erogenous zones. *Arch Sex Behav*. 45 (5). 1207-1216. DOI: 10.1007/s10508-016-0745-z

Younis, I. et al. (2016). Female hot spots: extragenital erogenous zones. *Hum Androl*. 6 (1). 20-26. DOI: 10.1097/01.XHA.0000481142.54302.08

92-93 What happens when we're aroused?
Masters, W. H. and Johnson, V. E. (1966). *Human sexual response*. US: Bantam Books.

Basson, R. (2001) Human sex-response cycles. *J Sex Marital Ther*. 27 (1). 33-43. DOI: 10.1080/00926230152035831

Chivers, M. L. et al. (2010). Agreement of self-reported and genital measures of sexual arousal in men and women *Arch Sex Behav*. 39 (1). 5-56. DOI: 10.1007/s10508-009-9556-9

94-95 How do erections happen?
Biga, L. M. et al. (2019). Physiology of arousal and orgasm. Anatomy and Physiology. Oregon State University. [online]. 1. 1864-72. https://open.oregonstate.education/aandp/chapter/27-5-physiology-of-arousal-and-orgasm/
Atomik Research Insights & Analytics. Co-op pharmacy erectile dysfunction PR Survey. [online]. www.atomikresearch.co.uk/case-studies-archive/co-op-pharmacy-erectile-dysfunction-pr-survey/
Davies, K. P. (2015). Development & therapeutic applications of nitric oxide releasing materials to treat erectile dysfunction. *Future Sci OA*. [online]. 1 (1). FSO53. DOI: 10.4155/fso.15.53
Shepherd Centre. Male Sexuality. [online]. www.myshepherdconnection.org/sci/sexuality/male-sexuality
Goldstein, I. The central mechanisms of sexual function. Boston University School of Medicine. [online]. www.bumc.bu.edu/sexualmedicine/publications/the-central-mechanisms-of-sexual-function/

96-97 What happens during orgasm?
Georgiadis, J. R. and Kringelbach, M. L. (2012). The human sexual response cycle: brain imaging evidence linking sex to other pleasures. *Progr neurobiol*. 98 (1). 49-81. DOI: 10.1016/j.pneurobio.2012.05.004
Stromberg, J. (2015). This is what your brain looks like during an orgasm. Vox. [online]. www.vox.com/2015/4/1/8325483/orgasms-science
Clarke, M. (2018). What's going on with hormones and neurotransmitters during sex. *Atlas Biomed*. [online]. https://atlasbiomed.com/blog/whats-going-on-with-hormones-and-neurotransmitters-during-sex/
Portner, M. (2008). The Orgasmic Mind: The neurological roots of sexual pleasure. *Scientific American*. [online]. www.scientificamerican.com/article/the-orgasmic-mind/
Wise, N. J., Komisaruk, B. R. et al. (2018). Brain activity unique to orgasm in women. *J Sex Med*. 14 (11). 1380–1391. DOI: 10.1016/j.jsxm.2017.08.014

98-99 Types of orgasm
Inverse. (2022). Why wearing socks during sex helps you have orgasms (online). www.inverse.com/mind-body/socks-sex-orgasms

100-101 Ejaculation/refractory period
ISSM's Communication Committee (2013). What is the refractory period? *ISSM*. [online]. www.issm.info/sexual-health-qa/what-is-the-refractory-period/

106-107 Menstrual cycle hormones
Lachowsky, M. and Nappi, R. E. (2009). The effect of oestrogen on urogenital health. *Maturitas*. 63 (2). 149-51. DOI: 10.1016/j.maturitas.2009.03.012
Chalabi, M. (2016). Going with the flow: how your period affects your sex drive. *The Guardian*. [online]. www.theguardian.com/lifeandstyle/2016/oct/15/how-period-affects-sex-drive-menstruation-ovulation

108-109 Testosterone
Wang, C. et al. (2011). Low testosterone associated with obesity and the metabolic syndrome contributes to sexual dysfunction and cardiovascular disease risk in men with type 2 diabetes. *Diabetes Care*. 34 (7). 1669-75. DOI: 10.2337/dc10-2339
Gettler, L. et al. (2011). Longitudinal evidence that fatherhood decreases testosterone in human males. *PNAS*. 108 (39). 16194-9. DOI: 10.1073/pnas.1105403108
Mount Sinai Today (2022). Testosterone. https://www.mountsinai.org/health-library/tests/testosterone
Marinov, D. (2022). Charts of average testosterone levels in male and female. *HFS Clinic*. [online]. https://hghfor-sale.com/blog/normal-testosterone-levels-by-age/

110-111 Love hormones
Wu, K. (2017). Love, actually: The science behind lust, attraction, and companionship. Harvard University. [online]. https://sitn.hms.harvard.edu/flash/2017/love-actually-science-behind-lust-attraction-companionship/
Owens, A. (2021). Tell me all I need to know about oxytocin. *Psycom*. [online]. www.psycom.net/oxytocin
Clarke, M. (2018). What's going on with hormones and neurotransmitters during sex. *Atlas Biomed*. [online]. https://atlasbiomed.com/blog/whats-going-on-with-hormones-and-neurotransmitters-during-sex/
Shoemaker, C. (2019). Male libido, testosterone, & neurotransmitters. *Sanesco*. [online]. https://sanescohealth.com/blog/male-libido-testosterone-nervous-system/

112-113 Pelvic floor exercises
Kanter, G. et al. (2015). A strong pelvic floor is associated with higher rates of sexual activity in women with pelvic floor disorders. *Int Urogynecol J*. 26 (7). 991-96. DOI: 10.1007/s00192-014-2583-7

116-117 Can I learn to love my body?
de Balzac, H. (2021). Scientific lessons to help you overcome self-doubt. Psychology Compass. [online]. https://psychologycompass.com/premium/self-doubt/
Cascio, C. N. (2015). Self-affirmation activates brain systems associated with self-related processing and reward and is reinforced by future orientation. *Soc Cogn Affect Neurosci*. 11 (4). DOI: 10.1093/scan/nsv136
Poirier, A. (2021). *The Body Joyful*. Woodhall Press.

118-119 Are sexual problems common?
Mitchell, K. R. et al. (2013). Sexual function in Britain: findings from the third national survey of sexual attitudes and lifestyles (Natsal-3). *Lancet*. [online] 382. 1817–29. www.natsal.ac.uk/sites/default/files/2021-04/Natsal-3%20infographics.pdf
BMJ Best Practice. Sexual dysfunction in women. [online]. https://bestpractice.bmj.com/topics/en-gb/352

120-121 Is painful sex normal?
Vaginismus (online). www.vaginismus.com/
The Gynae Centre (2021). Vaginismus: Debunking The Myths. The Gynae Centre Blog. [online]. www.gynae-centre.co.uk/blog/vaginismus-debunking-the-myths/

122-123 Erection problems
LetsGetChecked (2020). 3 in 5 men in US affected by erectile dysfunction. PR Newswire. [online]. www.prnewswire.com/news-releases/3-in-5-men-in-us-affected-by-erectile-dysfunction---and-most-are-unaware-it-can-be-an-indicator-of-more-serious-health-problems-301003952.html

128-129 Why does lust feel so intense?
Fisher, H. et al. (2002). Defining the brain systems of lust, romantic attraction and attachment. *Arch Sex Behav*, 31 (5). 413-9. DOI: 10.1023/a:1019888024255
NPR/TED staff (2019). Helen Fisher: How Does Love Affect The Brain? NPR. [online]. www.npr.org/2019/11/22/780960553/helen-fisher-how-does-love-affect-the-brain
Van Edwards, V. (2016). The 3 stages of love. Science of People. [online]. www.scienceofpeople.com/3-stages-of-love/
Wu, K. (2017). Love, actually: the science behind lust, attraction, and companionship. Harvard University. [online].

https://sitn.hms.harvard.edu/flash/2017/love-actually-science-behind-lust-attraction-companionship/
Gottman, J. (2014). The 3 phases of love. The Gottman Institute. [online]. www.gottman.com/blog/the-3-phases-of-love/

130-131 What happens when we feel desire?
Gurney, K. (2020). *Mind The Gap*. UK: Headline. p168.
Lifeworks (2017). What Basson's sexual response cycle teaches us about sexuality (online). www.lifeworkspsychotherapy.com/bassons-sexual-response-cycle-teaches-us-sexuality/

132-133 What are pheromones?
McClintock, M. K. (1971). Menstrual synchrony and suppression. *Nature*. 229. 244–45. DOI: 10.1038/229244a0
Verhaeghe, J. et al. (2013). Pheromones and their effect on women's mood and sexuality. *Facts, Views Vis ObGyn*. 5 (3). 189–95. PMID: 24753944

134-135 Aphrodisiacs
Eippert, F. (2009). Activation of the opioidergic descending pain control system underlies placebo analgesia. *Neuron*. 63 (4). 533-43. DOI: 10.1016/j.neuron.2009.07.014

136-137 Are we out of sync?
Brough, E. (2009). Positive emotions and sexual desire among healthy women. Research Gate. [online]. www.researchgate.net/publication/30863012
Mercer, C. H. et al. (2003). Sexual function problems and help seeking behaviour in Britain: National probability survey. *Br Med J*. 327. 426–427. DOI: 10.1136/bmj.327.7412.426
Mitchell, K. R. et al. (2013). Sexual function in Britain: findings from the third national survey of sexual attitudes and lifestyles (Natsal-3). *Lancet*. 382. 1817–1829. www.natsal.ac.uk/sites/default/files/2021-04/Natsal-3%20infographics.pdf

138-139 Does flirting improve sex?
Zhou, C. et al. (2018). Direct gaze blurs self-other boundaries. *J Gen Psychol*. 145 (3). 280-95. DOI: 10.1080/00221309.2018.1469465
Connole, S. (2019). Love: it's all in the eyes. Wholebeing Institute. [online]. https://wholebeinginstitute.com/love-its-all-in-the-eyes/
Jarick, M. and Bencic, R. (2019). Eye contact is a two-way street: arousal is elicited by the sending and receiving of eye gaze information. *Front Psychol*. 10 (1262). DOI: 10.3389/fpsyg.2019.01262
Nagasawa, M. (2015). Oxytocin-gaze positive loop and the coevolution of human-dog bonds. *Science*. 348 (6232). 333-36. DOI: 10.1126/science.1261022

140-141 Can novelty kindle desire?
Gurney, K. (2020). *Mind The Gap*. UK: Headline.

142-143 How do we connect?
Frederick, D. A. et al. (2016). What keeps passion alive? Sexual satisfaction is associated with sexual communication, mood setting, sexual variety, oral sex, orgasm and sex frequency in a national U.S. study. *J Sex Research*. 54 (2). 186-201. DOI: 10.1080/00224499.2015.1137854
Gillespie, B. J. (2016). Correlates of Sex Frequency and Sexual Satisfaction Among Partnered Older Adults. *J Sex Marit Ther*. 43 (5). DOI: 10.1080/0092623X.2016.1176608

144-145 What's a fetish?
Pfeuffer, R. (2023). A list of 25 sexual kinks and fetishes we know you're curious about. Men's Health. [online]. www.menshealth.com/sex-women/a33338854/kinks-fetish-list/

149 Holiday sex
Kalmbach, D. A. et al. (2015). The impact of sleep on female sexual response and behavior. *J Sex Med*. 12 (5). 1221–32. DOI: 10.1111/jsm.12858

150-151 Best time of day for sex
Barberia, J. M. et al. (1973). Diurnal variations of plasma testosterone in men. *Steroids*. 22 (5). 615-626. DOI: 10.1016/0039-128X(73)90110-4

152-153 Are phones in the way?
This Works (2020). Love sleep report. https://viewer.joomag.com/love-sleep-report-final-2020-love-sleep-report-final/0922298001580726302?

154-155 Can a sex break reboot desire?
Trigwell, P. et al. (2015). The Leeds psychosexual medicine service: an NHS service for sexual dysfunction. *Sex Relation Ther*. 31 (1). 32-41. DOI: 10.1080/14681994.2015.1078459
Linschoten, M. et al. (2016). Sensate focus: a critical literature review. *Sex Relation Ther*. 31 (2). 230-47. DOI: 10.1080/14681994.2015.1127909

158-159 What turns us on and off?
Dee, J. (2016). The dual control model – Why you sometimes can't get in the mood for sex. Uncovering Intimacy. [online]. www.uncoveringintimacy.com/dual-control-model-sometimes-cant-get-mood-sex/
Map Education and Research Foundation. The history of the sexual tipping point® model. [online]. www.mapedfund.org/history
Bancroft, J. and Janssen, E. (2000). The dual control model of male sexual response: a theoretical approach to centrally mediated erectile dysfunction. *Neurosci Biobehav Rev* 24 (5). 571-79. DOI: 10.1016/s0149-7634(00)00024-5
Kinsey Institute. Dual control model of sexual response. [online]. https://kinseyinstitute.org/research/dual-control-model.php

160-161 Arousal non-concordance
Embrace Sexual Wellness (2020). Arousal non concordance. ESW Blog. [online]. www.embracesexualwellness.com/esw-blog/arousalnonconcordance
Jean-Baptiste, O. (2021). The common sexual health issue you probably didn't know about. The Zoe Report. [online]. www.thezoereport.com/wellness/what-is-arousal-non-concordance
Chivers, M. L. et al. (2010). Agreement of self-reported and genital measures of sexual arousal in men and women. *Arch Sex Behav*. 39 (1). 5-56. DOI: 10.1007/s10508-009-9556-9
Brotto, L. A. et al. (2016) Mindfulness-based sex therapy improves genital-subjective arousal concordance in women with sexual desire/arousal difficulties. *Arch Sex Behav*. 45 (8). 1907-1921. DOI: 0.1007/s10508-015-0689-8
Chivers, M. L. and Brotto. L. A. (2017). Controversies of women's sexual arousal and desire. *Euro Psychol*. 22 (1). 5-26. DOI: 10.1027/1016-9040/a000274

162-163 Good conditions for sex
Gurney, K. (2020). *Mind The Gap*. UK: Headline.

164-165 Who initiates sex
Lehmiller, J. (2018). *Tell me what you want: the science of sexual desire and how it can help you improve your sex life*. Robinson.

166 Avoiding feelings of rejection
Meston, C. M. and Buss, D.M. (2007) Why humans have sex. *Arch Sex Behav*. [online]. 36. 477-507. https://labs.la.utexas.edu/mestonlab/files/2016/05/WhyHaveSex.pdf

170–171 The orgasm gap
Frederick, D.A. et al. (2018). Differences in orgasm frequency among gay, lesbian, bisexual, and heterosexual men and women in a U.S. national sample. *Arch Sex Behav* 47, 273–88. DOI: 10.1007/s10508-017-0939-z
Mintz, Laurie. B. (2017). Becoming cliterate: why orgasm equality matters and how to get it. HarperOne, Harper Collins.
Kinsey, A. et al. (1953). *Sexual Behavior in the Human Female.* Philadelphia: W. B. Saunders.

172–173 Does faking it matter?
Herbenick, D. et al. (2019). Women's sexual satisfaction, communication, and reasons for (no longer) faking orgasm: findings from a U.S. probability sample. *Arch Sex Behav.* DOI: 10.1007/s10508-019-01493-0
Muehlenhard, C. L. and Shippee, S. K. (2010). Men's and women's reports of pretending orgasm. *J Sex Res.* 47 (6). 552-67. DOI: 10.1080/00224490903171794.
Ballard, J. (2022). Women are more likely than men to say they're a people-pleaser. YouGov America. [online]. https://today.yougov.com/topics/society/articles-reports/2022/08/22/women-more-likely-men-people-pleasing-poll

176-177 Why does talking about sex feel taboo?
Ramírez-Villalobos, D. et al. (2021). Delaying sexual onset: outcome of a comprehensive sexuality education initiative for adolescents in public schools. *BMC Public Health.* 21 (1439). DOI: 10.1186/s12889-021-11388-2
Peanut and Headspace (2021). Your sexual wellness isn't taboo. [online] www.peanut-app.io/blog/peanut-headspace-sexual-wellness-for-women

180-183 Mindful sex
Brotto, l. (2018). *Better Sex Through Mindfulness: How Women Can Cultivate Desire.* Greystone Books Ltd
Hamilton, L. D. et al. (2008). Cortisol, sexual arousal and affect in response to sexual stimuli. *J Sex Med.* 5 (9). 2111–8. DOI: 10.1111/j.1743-6109.2008.00922.x
Goyal, M. et al. (2014). Meditation Programs for Psychological Stress and Well-being. *JAMA Intern Med.* 174(3): 357–368. DOI:10.1001/jamainternmed.2013.13018

186-187 Is sexuality fluid?
Kinsey, A. C. et al. (1948/1998). *Sexual Behavior in the Human Male.* Philadelphia: W. B. Saunders; Bloomington: Indiana U. Press. [Kinsey's Heterosexual-Homosexual Scale, 636–659.]

194-195 Sexual health
World Health Organization. Sexual health. [online]. www.who.int/health-topics/sexual-health#tab=tab_2

198-201 Protection/contraception
NHS. Your contraception guide. [online]. www.nhs.uk/conditions/contraception/

204-205 STIs
World Health Organization. Sexually transmitted infections (STIs). [online]. www.who.int/news-room/fact-sheets/detail/sexually-transmitted-infections-(stis)
Centers for Disease Control and Prevention. Genital HPV Infection – Basic Fact Sheet. [online]. www.cdc.gov/std/hpv/stdfact-hpv.htm
NHS. HPV vaccine overview. [online]. www.nhs.uk/conditions/vaccinations/hpv-human-papillomavirus-vaccine/
Vaccine Knowledge. HPV Vaccine (Human Papillomavirus Vaccine). [online]. https://vk.ovg.ox.ac.uk/hpv-vaccine#The-impact-of-the-HPV-programme

Centers for Disease Control and Prevention. HPV Vaccine Safety and Effectiveness. [online]. www.cdc.gov/vaccines/vpd/hpv/hcp/safety-effectiveness.html

206-207 Sexual health screening
Pebody, R. (2021). What is the window period for HIV testing? NAM. [online]. www.aidsmap.com/about-hiv/what-window-period-hiv-testing

210-211 Sexual trauma
Bremner, J. D. (2006). Traumatic stress: effects on the brain. *Dialogues Clin Neurosci.* 8 (4). 445-61. DOI: 10.31887/DCNS.2006.8.4/jbremner
Elzinga, B. M. and Bremner, J. D. (2002). Are the neural substrates of memory the final common pathway in posttraumatic stress disorder (PTSD)? *J Affect Disord.* 70 (1). 1-17. DOI: 10.1016/s0165-0327(01)00351-2
Yoon, S.A.and Weierich, M.R. Persistent amygdala novelty response is associated with less anterior cingulum integrity in trauma-exposed women. *Neuroimage Clin.* 2017 Jan 16; 14: 250-259. DOI: 10.1016/j.nicl.2017.01.015

220-221 Bids for attention
Lisitsa, E. (2012). An introduction to emotional bids and trust. The Gottman Institute. [online]. www.gottman.com/blog/an-introduction-to-emotional-bids-and-trust/

225 Sexting
Holmes, L. G. (2021). A sex-positive mixed methods approach to sexting experiences among college students. *Comput Hum Behav.* 115. DOI: 10.1016/j.chb.2020.106619
McNichols, N. K. (2021). Some surprising benefits of sexting in a relationship. Psychology Today. [online]. www.psychologytoday.com/gb/blog/everyone-top/202106/some-surprising-benefits-sexting-in-relationship

227 Rebuilding sexual confidence
Eisenberger, N. I. (2012). Broken hearts and broken bones: a neural perspective on the similarities between social and physical pain. *Current Directions in Psychol Sci.* 21 (1). 42–47. DOI: 10.1177/0963721411429455

228-229 Sex over time
Relate (2018). Over a quarter of relationships are 'sexless'. [online]. www.relate.org.uk/get-help/over-quarter-relationships-are-sexless

230-231 Sex after a baby
NHS. Sex and contraception after birth. [online]. www.nhs.uk/conditions/baby/support-and-services/sex-and-contraception-after-birth/
Extend Fertility. Fertility Statistics by Age. [online]. https://extendfertility.com/your-fertility/fertility-statistics-by-age/
La Leche League International. Breastfeeding and sex. [online]. www.llli.org/breastfeeding-info/breastfeeding-and-sex/

232-233 Genitals ageing
Vinmec. How does the penis change with age? [online]. www.vinmec.com/en/news/health-news/healthy-lifestyle/how-does-the-penis-change-with-age/

234-235 Menopause
NHS. Menopause. [online]. www.nhs.uk/conditions/menopause/

Index

Data credits

The publisher would like to thank the following for their kind permission to reproduce their data:
p.65: Lehmiller, J. (2018). *Tell Me What You Want: The Science of Sexual Desire and How It Can Help You Improve Your Sex Life*. Robinson. p.131. Data from Rose.
p.131: Rosemary Basson. (2001). Female sexual response: the role of drugs in the management of sexual dysfunction, *Obstet and Gynecol*, 98 (2), 2001. 350-353, ISSN 0029-7844. DOI:10.1016/S0029-7844(01)01452-1.
p.161: Chivers M. L., et al. (2010) Agreement of self-reported and genital measures of sexual arousal in men and women: a meta-analysis. *Arch Sex Behav*. Feb; 39 (1): 5-56. DOI: 10.1007/s10508-009-9556-9.
p.170: Frederick, D.A., et al. (2018). Differences in orgasm frequency among gay, lesbian, bisexual, and heterosexual men and women in a U.S. national sample. *Arch Sex Behav*. 47: 273-288. DOI: 10.1007/s10508-017-0939-z
p.221: The Gottman Institute: https://www.gottman.com/blog/turn-toward-instead-of-away/
p.225: Laura Graham Holmes, A. Renee Nilssen, Deanna Cann, Donald S. Strassberg. (2021). A sex-positive mixed methods approach to sexting experiences among college students, *Computers in Human Behavior*, V 115. 106619. DOI: 10.1016/j.chb.2020.106619

Acknowledgments

About the author

Kate Moyle is a psychosexual and relationship therapist, EFS-ESSM certified psycho-sexologist, and host of *The Sexual Wellness Sessions* podcast. She works in talking therapy to help people address the challenges they're facing in their sex lives and relationships, and to help people get to a place of sexual health, wellbeing, and happiness, whatever that looks like for them. She wholeheartedly believes in the power of education and conversation to change our culture around sex for the better. She holds a degree in Psychology, a diploma in Integrative Psychosexual Therapy and a Masters in Relationship Therapy. Kate takes her knowledge and learning from inside the therapy room to work with brands and the media as an expert consultant on the subject of sexual wellness, and is a regular guest on panels, podcasts, in the media, and at events. You can find Kate at: www.katemoyle.co.uk; on Instagram: @KateMoyleTherapy; and listen to Kate on *The Sexual Wellness Sessions* podcast.

Author's acknowledgments

While I've always known I wanted to write a book on the topic of sex, I hadn't formulated an idea of what that would look like until I was approached by Zara Anvari at DK. Given that one of the biggest parts of my job is asking questions and helping people to find their own answers, I hope that this book reflects so many of the questions that a lot of us have about sex across our lifetimes.

My first thanks goes to Cabby Laffy, founder and teacher of my psychosexual therapy training at The Centre For Psychosexual Health, London. Her open-mindedness and words from the day she offered me a place on the training remain etched in my memory, and it's where my love for this work really began.

To colleagues and supervisors, past and present, for sharing their wisdom; I've learnt something from each and every one of you. Particular mention to Silva Neves for his continuous support always, but especially on this book, alongside those who've allowed me to pick their minds along the writing way - Catriona Boffard, Aoife Drury, Clare Faulkner, Dr Naomi Sutton, Julie Sale, and Dr Sarah Welsh.

Thank you for allowing me my questions and using you for reassurance and clarity.

To anyone who has ever sat across from me in the therapy chair, I'll never doubt how hard booking and attending that initial appointment can be, and how challenging therapy can feel. My job is a privilege and I learn something new about human sexuality from every person I work with. So much of sex is nuanced and can only be fully understood through people and their experiences; this part of our understanding of sex can't be academically taught.

And personally, for the support from home, family, and friends, without which I could do none of what I do. One person's time can only be split so many ways and everyone has played a part in getting this book from ideas to bookshelf. There are many people who've made the different parts of my life possible, and I could not have done it without the moral, physical, childcare, and emotional support. Particular thanks to my parents and family who've supported me from day one and always helped me get to where I wanted to go; and my husband, who always encourages my ideas and ambitions, even when he knows there's always a next one, and that a therapist's learning is never done. For everything, thank you.

And for my children, nieces, nephews, godchildren, and all the future generations - I hope that this plays a small part in shifting your sexual culture for the better.

Another huge thank you is owed to the others who've worked so hard to bring this book to life. At DK, Becky Alexander, Glenda Fisher, and Izzy Holton. Particular thanks to Claire Cross, the editor of this book, without whom it would not exist and for her unlimited patience and curiosity, and to designers Emma and Tom Forge and Jocelyn Covarrubias, our amazing illustrator.

About the illustrator

Jocelyn Covarrubias is an artist who enjoys celebrating women's mental health, body norms, sexuality, and everyday life through minimalistic art in order to provide people with a sense of belonging and confidence in their own skin. She is based in New York and her work can be found on Instagram: @joce_cova.

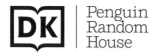

Senior Acquisitions Editor Zara Anvari, Becky Alexander
Project Editor Izzy Holton
Senior Designers Glenda Fisher, Louise Brigenshaw
Editorial Assistant Charlotte Beauchamp
Production Editor David Almond
Production Controller Luca Bazzoli
Jacket Designer Amy Cox
Jacket Co-ordinator Jasmin Lennie
Editorial Manager Ruth O'Rourke
Art Director Maxine Pedliham
Publishing Director Katie Cowan

Editor Claire Cross
Design Emma Forge, Tom Forge
Styling Sarah Pyke
Illustration Jocelyn Covarrubias

First published in Great Britain in 2023 by
Dorling Kindersley Limited
DK, One Embassy Gardens, 8 Viaduct Gardens,
London, SW11 7BW

The authorised representative in the EEA is
Dorling Kindersley Verlag GmbH. Arnulfstr. 124,
80636 Munich, Germany

A CIP catalogue record for this book
is available from the British Library.
ISBN: 978-0-2415-9329-5

Printed and bound in China

For the curious
www.dk.com

MIX
Paper | Supporting
responsible forestry
FSC™ C018179
www.fsc.org

This book was made with Forest
Stewardship Council ™ certified
paper - one small step in DK's
commitment to a sustainable future.
**For more information go to
www.dk.com/our-green-pledge**

DK would like to thank Dr Kit Heyam for
the sensitivity read; Claire Wedderburn-
Maxwell for proofreading; and Hilary Bird
for the index.

Disclaimer

The information in this book has been
compiled by way of general guidance in
relation to the specific subjects addressed.
It is not a substitute and not to be relied on
for medical, healthcare, pharmaceutical,
or other professional advice on specific
circumstances and in specific locations.
Please consult your GP before starting,
changing, or stopping any medical
treatment. So far as the author is aware,
the information given is correct and up
to date as of March 2023. Practice, laws,
and regulations all change, and the reader
should obtain up-to-date professional
advice on any such issues. The naming of
any product, treatment, or organization in
this book does not imply endorsement
by the author or publisher, nor does the
omission of any such names indicate
disapproval. The author and publisher
disclaim, as far as the law allows, any
liability arising directly or indirectly from
the use, or misuse, of the information
contained in this book.

A note on gender identities

DK recognizes all gender identities, and
acknowledges that the sex someone was
assigned at birth based on their sexual
organs may not align with their own
gender identity. People may self-identify
as any gender or no gender (including,
but not limited to, that of a cis or trans
woman, of a cis or trans man, or of a
non-binary person).

As gender language, and its use in our
society, evolves, the scientific and medical
communities continue to reassess their own
phrasing. Most of the studies referred to in
this book use "women" to describe people
whose sex was assigned as female at birth,
and "men" to describe people whose sex
was assigned as male at birth.